ADVANCE PRAISE FOR
HOW TO MANAGE PAIN IN THE ELDERLY

"*How to Manage Pain in the Elderly* provides an overview of pain assessment instruments, evidence-based pain management strategies, and pain management considerations at the end of life. This book is a nice addition to a growing body of literature that will assist nurses in providing more effective pain management to the older population."

–Meredith Wallace, PhD, APRN
Associate Professor
Yale University School of Nursing

"This comprehensive text exposes myths about pain management in seniors. It goes well beyond pain as the fifth vital sign by focusing our attention on the complexities and key issues in improving the quality of pain management in older adults. *How to Manage Pain in the Elderly* provides readers a critical analysis of the evidence; supplies details about dosages and drug potency; and highlights often-overlooked aspects of pain in terminal patients, nonverbal patients, and community-living older adults. The author also addresses the important issues of which drugs to avoid and what side effects pain medications may cause. This book presents a practical and multifaceted approach to improving pain management in older adults. It is long overdue."

–Donna M. Fick, PhD, GCNS-BC, FAAN
Associate Professor
School of Nursing and College of Medicine
The Pennsylvania State University

D1559467

HOW TO
MANAGE
PAIN
IN THE *Elderly*

Yvonne D'Arcy, MS, CRNP, CNS

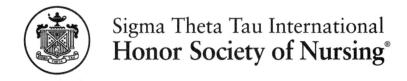

Sigma Theta Tau International
Honor Society of Nursing®

Sigma Theta Tau International
550 West North Street
Indianapolis, IN 46202

To order additional books, buy in bulk, or order for corporate use, contact Nursing Knowledge International at 888.NKI.4YOU (888.654.4968/US and Canada) or +1.317.634.8171 (outside US and Canada).

To request a review copy for course adoption, e-mail solutions@nursingknowledge.org or call 888.NKI.4YOU (888.654.4968/US and Canada) or +1.317.917.4983 (outside US and Canada).

To request author information, or for speaker or other media requests, contact Rachael McLaughlin of the Honor Society of Nursing, Sigma Theta Tau International at 888.634.7575 (US and Canada) or +1.317.634.8171 (outside US and Canada).

ISBN-13: 978-1-930538-84-9

Library of Congress Cataloging-in-Publication Data

D'Arcy, Yvonne M.
  How to manage pain in the elderly / Yvonne D'Arcy.
    p. ; cm.
  Includes bibliographical references and index.
  ISBN 978-1-930538-84-9
  1. Pain in old age--Treatment. I. Sigma Theta Tau International. II. Title.
  [DNLM: 1. Geriatric Nursing--methods. 2. Pain--nursing. 3. Aged. 4. Pain--therapy. 5. Palliative Care--methods. WY 152 D214h 2010]
  RB127.D377 2010
  618.97'0231--dc22
                        2009047776

First Printing, 2009

Publisher: Renee Wilmeth
Acquisitions Editor: Cynthia Saver, RN, MS
Development Editor: John Sleeva
Production Editor: Billy Fields

Copy Editor and Proofreader: Jane Palmer
Editorial Coordinator: Paula Jeffers
Indexer: Angie Bess Martin, RN
Cover Design by: Rebecca Batchelor
Illustrator: Rebecca Batchelor

DEDICATION

To all the health care providers who are caring for older patients, my thanks for helping these wonderful patients with their pain management needs. I hope you will find this book helpful in your endeavors, and I wish you much success in treating the pain of your elderly patients.

About the Author

Yvonne D'Arcy, MS, CRNP, CNS, is the pain management and palliative care nurse practitioner at Suburban Hospital, Johns Hopkins Medicine, Bethesda, Maryland. She has worked more than 14 years as an advanced practice nurse with a specialty in pain management. She received her master's degree in 1995 from Winona State University in Minnesota and her nurse practitioner certificate from the University of Florida in 1999. In addition, she has pursued doctoral studies at the University of Florida and the University of Maryland in Baltimore.

D'Arcy has served on the board of directors for the American Society of Pain Management Nurses and is a member of the American Pain Society and the American Academy of Nurse Practitioners. In 2005, D'Arcy was voted Advanced Practice Nurse of the Year at Suburban Hospital, and she was district winner of the *Nursing Spectrum* Nursing Excellence Award in 2007 for the category of Advancing and Leading the Profession. She was coordinator of the Acute Pain Service and supervisor of the Chronic Pain Clinic at Mayo Clinic in Jacksonville, Florida, from 1996 to 2001. She moved to Baltimore, Maryland, to work as coordinator of the Oncology Pain Service for Johns Hopkins Oncology Center.

Her current position allows her to combine the practice of pain management with palliative care.

D'Arcy writes and presents nationally on various pain management topics, including chronic pain, pain assessment, difficult-to-treat neuropathic pain syndromes, pain in addicted patients, and pain in older patients. She is the recipient of the Gold Award for best "how-to series" from the American Society of Healthcare Publications Editors for A Field Guide to Pain Management. In 2007, D'Arcy published her first book, *Pain Management: Evidence-Based Tools and Techniques for Nursing Professionals.* She is a frequent contributor to the Pain Solutions column in the *Journal for Nurse Practitioners.* In addition, she has written numerous articles for journals and chapters for nursing textbooks.

Table of Contents

1 THE AGING OF AMERICA:
  THE PROBLEM OF PAIN IN OLDER
  ADULTS............................. 1

2 PAIN ASSESSMENT IN THE OLDER
  PATIENT 11

3 PAIN MEDICATION MANAGEMENT
  FOR OLDER ADULTS 33

4 COMPLEMENTARY METHODS FOR
  PAIN RELIEF........................ 61

5 ACUTE PAIN MANAGEMENT............ 77

6 CHRONIC PAIN MANAGEMENT......... 95

7 INTERVENTIONAL PAIN MANAGEMENT
  FOR OLDER PATIENTS................ 121

8 PALLIATIVE CARE................... 143

  REFERENCES....................... 165

  INDEX............................ 177

INTRODUCTION

For most people, aging is part of the human condition. Unfortunately, pain is also likely at some point in life. Individuals who have never had pain from surgery, injury, or a chronic condition are lucky, and rare. A select few, because of genetics, cannot feel pain, but most people have experienced some type of pain, and most have found the experience to be negative.

For the older patient, pain may be considered as part of life. However, pain in older patients can be treated with medications, interventional options, and complementary techniques. When pain is not adequately treated in older patients, they may avoid social contact, become isolated and depressed, and suffer sleep disturbances. Unrelieved pain in older patients has a negative impact on their quality of life.

Many health care practitioners I meet are afraid of using opioids for pain in older patients. They fear the patient will become over-sedated and the medications will cause other adverse effects, such as nausea, vomiting, or constipation. I would refer these well-meaning health care providers to one of our octogenarian pain-service patients. She vociferously refused to return to her nursing home after we started her on a very low dose of an opioid, which reduced her pain significantly. She said that we were the ones who understood her pain best. Using the right dose of the right pain medication and providing safe prescribing practices with regular monitoring parameters can allow older patients to return to a meaningful, productive lifestyle.

This book is designed to provide helpful and usable clinical information about pain in the older patient. Topics include information on medications, pain assessment, and effects of certain difficult-to-treat pain conditions that affect older patients. Each chapter has a case study with questions designed to help the reader use the information provided in the chapter. Clinical pearls have been inserted into the text of each chapter to highlight important considerations for treatment or to provide additional information. A chapter with helpful information on using complementary techniques is included for providers who are interested in complementary methods for relieving pain. And finally, as chronic illness progresses, many older patients will need to consider palliative care; the last chapter contains some salient information on symptom management in palliative care.

1

THE AGING OF AMERICA: THE PROBLEM OF PAIN IN OLDER ADULTS

Aging is defined as a progressive, generalized impairment of function, resulting in the loss of adaptive response to stress and in a growing risk of age-related disease (Hadjistavropoulos et al., 2007). The aging of a population results in an increased need for health care based on increased age-related diseases. Because many of these diseases are painful, there is an increased need for pain management. Chronic diseases such as osteoarthritis, diabetic neuropathy, degenerative back disease, and other neuropathic syndromes can all cause pain that may limit function and decrease quality of life for the older patient.

In addition to the results of chronic illness, older patients face loss of independence and functionality when they become less able to care for themselves and become more physically impaired. Statistics indicate that the proportion of Americans who are 65 years of age or older has tripled the past 100 years, and the life expectancy has increase from 47 years in 1900 to 77.2 years in 2001 (Smeltzer, Bare, Hinkle, & Cheever, 2008). By 2030, one in five United States citizens (about 70 million people) will be 65 or older (Smeltzer et al., 2008). The very old population will increase as well. In 2002 there were 50,564 people 100 years of age or older, an increase of 35% from 1900 (Smeltzer et al.).

CATEGORIZING THE OLDER PATIENT

- **Younger old:** 65 to 75 years of age. The number in this group is 7% of the total population.

- **Older old:** 75 to 84 years of age. The number in this group is 4% of the total population.

- **Elite old:** 85 years of age or older. This group is 1% of the total population (AHCA, 2009).

These statistics indicate that the percentage of patients in the older old and elite old age groups is likely to increase in future years. Patients will be living longer and need more assistance as they age.

Overall, it is estimated that 43% of the people who turned 65 in 1990 will enter a nursing home at some time in their lives (AHCA, 2009). There are approximately 1.5 million nursing home residents in the United States (AHCA, 2009). Additional information indicates that 50% of patients in nursing homes suffer from untreated pain (AHCA, 2009). The 2002 American Geriatrics Society (AGS) paper on persistent pain in older patients reported that 45% to 80% of patients in long-term care had chronic daily pain.

Pain is also quite significant for older people who live in the community. Between 25% and 50% of community-dwelling older patients have chronic pain that may impair their ability to function (AGS, 2002). Undertreated or untreated pain has many negative consequences for older patients, including

- Depression

- Anxiety

- Decreased socialization

- Disturbed sleep

- Impaired ambulation

- Increased health care utilization and subsequent costs

- Impaired cognition

- Altered nutrition

  (D'Arcy, 2007; Bruckenthal & D'Arcy, 2007; AGS, 2002)

Some of the untreated pain is related to the fact that older patients, in general, do not like to take medication. If financial resources are limited, older patients may decide to endure the pain rather than spend money needed for household expenses on medication. This financial concern has reached into everyday clinical practice. In a recent survey of 400 nurse practitioners, when ranking barriers to prescribing opioid medications for their patients, respondents indicated that cost was their number one barrier (D'Arcy, 2009b).

MYTHS ABOUT PAIN AND THE OLDER PATIENT

Several myths surround pain and treating pain in the older adult, including

- Pain is a normal part of aging.

- Older patients cannot tolerate opioid medications.

- Older patients do not feel pain in the same way that younger patients do.

- Cognitively impaired patients do not experience pain.

If the patient does not report pain, it does not exist (Bruckenthal & D'Arcy, 2007; D'Arcy, 2009a).

Let's look at these misperceptions and see what can be substantiated.

- **Is pain a normal part of aging?** Pain is not a normal part of aging, although older patients do have a higher number of painful comorbidities, such as diabetic neuropathies, osteoarthritis, fractures and injuries from falls, compression fractures from osteoporosis, and impaired circulation. There are, of course, older patients who do not have pain or painful conditions. Because older patients may not access health care for their pain needs, they may be overlooked in the larger picture of the older patient population.

- **Can older patients tolerate opioid medications?** Yes, older patients can tolerate opioid medications, but the process of medication initiation and dosing needs to be carefully considered and monitored (AGS, 2002). The recommendation is to start low and go slow, reducing the normal opioid doses by 25% to 50% for older patients (McLennon, 2005). Because older patients may be more sensitive to adverse drug reactions, opioid medications should be started with careful monitoring on a trial basis, to see if they are effective in relieving pain. If the medication is effective and adverse effects are not significant, a pain relief regimen that includes opioids can be very beneficial for the patient. Placebos should never be used to determine whether the patient's pain is real, or to replace pain medication (AGS, 2002; American Pain Society [APS], 2008; D'Arcy, 2007). Using placebos destroys the patient's trust in the health care provider and has moral and legal implications for practice. Trying a placebo, which might be

> **Under Advisement**
>
> *Opioid Toxicity*
> With older patients who have decreased liver and kidney functions, opioid medication can take a longer time to be excreted. Decreasing doses will help to reduce the potential for opioid toxicity (McLennon, 2005).

considered a "safer" option, will only result in untreated and undertreated pain.

- **Does pain sensation decrease as patients age?** The results on this topic are mixed. Although patients' pain pathways do not change dramatically over time, comorbidities that patients develop as they age can affect the pain transmission process. For example, diabetes can lead to diabetic neuropathies in a stocking–glove distribution (feet and hands), where nerves are damaged by years of high blood sugar levels. Neuropathies and other conditions can also affect the older patient's ability to maintain a steady gait and balance. When an older patient with a comorbidity such as diabetes or cardiac disease is taking opioids, safety concerns must be addressed to decrease the potential for falls.

- **Do cognitively impaired patients experience pain?** Cognitive impairment also impedes perception of a sensation as pain. The cognitively impaired patient experiences pain along the same pain pathways as other patients. But, the cognitively impaired individual may not identify the sensation as pain. The difficulty with assessing pain in this group of patients adds to the complexity of the situation. There are now several pain assessment tools designed for cognitively impaired or nonverbal patients that rely on pain behaviors. Using one of these tools consistently can help the caregiver determine if the patient is in pain and if so, trigger administration of pain medication.

- **Why would a patient not report pain?** An older patient might choose not to report pain for several reasons. For example, if the older patient has cancer, increasing pain may signal a progression of the disease that is not the expected or wanted outcome. For other patients, the cost of tests and medications may be too prohibitive for them to consider reporting the pain. Still others may not like the way pain medications make them feel. For example, patients may stop pain medication without telling their doctor because the medication makes them feel "fuzzy-headed"; they would rather experience pain than be unable to think clearly.

The myths about pain medication and older patients really are that: myths. Older patients can tolerate pain medications, but prescribers may be unsure what to order and how to dose the medication to avoid adverse effects. In reality, if the pain remains untreated or undertreated, the effect can be far more damaging to the patient. Health care providers who see older patients should become familiar with reducing opioid doses, monitoring responses, and treating side effects such as constipation.

The Effect of the Older Patient's Physiology on Pain Medication Use

The older patient brings a very experienced body to the use of pain medications. Over the years, the patient may have used medication to relieve the pain of surgery, injuries such as sprains and strains, neuropathic conditions, or just plain headaches. As the body ages, it changes in ways that affect the metabolism of pain medication.

Changes in medication metabolism fall into the following four categories:

- **Absorption:** Medication may be absorbed more slowly in older patients because of increased gastric pH, decreased intestinal blood flow, and delayed gastric emptying.

- **Distribution:** Drugs can remain longer in the tissues, which increases time for action. This change is due to a decrease in lean body mass and total body water in older patients, as well as an increase in body fat and plasma protein. Lipid solubility and protein binding are directly affected by these changes.

- **Changed metabolism:** Clearance of medications and medication half-life are extended because of decreased liver mass, decreased microsomal enzyme activity, and decreased hepatic blood flow in older patients.

- **Excretion and elimination:** Most medications are excreted renally. Older patients have decreased glomerular filtration rate, decreased creatinine clearance, and decreased renal blood. These changes delay the elimination of medications (Bruckenthal & D'Arcy, 2007; St. Marie, 2002).

With all the changes that take place in the older patient's physiology, it is important to take a good history and perform lab tests, a physical examination, and a baseline functionality screen when medications are first prescribed. Determining the patient's ability to follow instructions for the medication and take medications as prescribed is also important. Pill boxes can be helpful here, as well as pill counts when the patient brings the medications to the clinic visit.

SUMMARY

The increase in the number of older patients will surely require a higher focus on treating pain in older patients. Addressing the myths and concerns of the older patient can help decrease the potential for undertreating pain in this particularly vulnerable population. As science progresses in its understanding of the physiology of aging, medications can be tailored to fit the needs of the older patient population. A dedicated health care team is essential to effective pain treatment, especially if opioids are used. Treating pain effectively, and thus preserving the patient's quality of life, can be a most gratifying clinical success.

CASE STUDY

Each chapter will include a case study to review concepts covered in the chapter. This first case study is based on concepts presented in the medication and assessment chapters. However, it can be used as a tool for understanding the types of questions that should be asked when problem-solving pain management issues in the older patient.

Peter Jones is a 79-year-old man who resides in an assisted living facility. He has a variety of comorbidities, including diabetes, hypertension, osteoarthritis, and mild memory problems. In the past, he has fallen and broken his hip and wrist. He takes 20 medications every day, including a vitamin supplement and some over-the-counter medications.

Peter is having difficulty remembering to take his medications, and he tells his physician that he has back pain and pain in his knees. The staff at the assisted living facility reports that Peter has become less social and stays in his room more. Occasionally, he wanders the halls at night. When the staff questions him the next morning, he does not remember leaving his apartment.

You are seeing Peter because he has fallen again and has an intense, sharp pain in his back that is localized and does not radiate. He moans and tells you, "I hurt right there. Please help me; I can't stand the pain." The MRI reveals that Peter has a compression fracture of two thoracic vertebrae.

Critical Analysis Questions

1. What is the best method to assess Peter's pain?

2. What would be the best option for medication to treat Peter's pain?

3. Is there an interventional pain-relief option that would help Peter's pain?

4. Can you start opioid medication to help the pain?

5. Should you consider any complementary methods for pain control?

6. Does Peter's osteoarthritis influence his present acute pain?

7. What are some of the biggest considerations about Peter and his pain, discharge planning, and medication administration?

2

PAIN ASSESSMENT IN THE OLDER PATIENT

Assessing the pain of older patients can present more of a challenge than assessing the pain of younger patients, simply because older patients may require more time and need more education on how to use a pain scale. Or, they may have barriers such as vision, hearing, or cognitive deficits. Furthermore, some older patients fear reporting pain or increased pain. This may be related to the following factors:

- The fear that a disease may be progressing: More pain might mean more disease. This may be particularly true for cancer patients or patients with other chronic, painful illnesses.

- Perceived threats to independent living. The patient may think, "If the pain increases, I will not be able to live alone or in my apartment."

- Threats to self-esteem and personal worth. "I can't feel good about myself if I admit I have pain every day."

- The desire to be a "good patient" and not complain about something they feel may have no solution.

- Thinking that pain is a normal part of aging, and they are just getting old.

To perform a meaningful pain assessment on older adults, the nurse must create an environment of trust, where patients feel comfortable talking about their pain. The assessment should include a discussion of how the pain affects patients' daily lives. Will they be able to continue living alone, or will they need more support for daily living activities? Can some aspects of daily life, such as meal preparation, be taken over by a church program or a community program such as Meals on Wheels? Can the patients go to a community center for a meal, not only to enjoy the meal but also the companionship of other older community members?

Assessing pain in older patients requires more time and effort by the health care provider. Some older patients feel that the nurse should just know they are in pain, without having to be told. These patients should be reassured that the reason the nurse is asking about the pain is because he or she is interested in helping to relieve the pain. Nurses are in an ideal situation to help all members of the health care team understand the pain an older patient is reporting. The use of therapeutic communication techniques, such as being present, active listening, and reflection, can help the patient relax and feel less threatened about reporting pain levels. For nonverbal patients or those with cognitive impairment or dementia, special assessment methods and scales should be used to determine if the patient is having pain.

Assessment Elements and Essentials

When assessing a patient's pain, it is important to get as much information as possible. An accurate judgment of the pain and its impact on the patient is essential in developing a suitable plan of care. All pain assessments should include the following basic elements:

- **Location:** Have the patient point to the place that is painful. If the patient cannot reach the location, place your hand in the area and palpate softly until you locate the site of the pain. Confirm with the patient that this is the painful area. If there are several areas, ask which one is most painful or has the biggest impact on function or sleep, and focus more attention on that area.

- **Intensity:** To determine pain intensity, a simple Likert-type pain scale such as the Numeric Pain Intensity (NPI), also called the Numeric Rating Scale (NRS), is most useful. To guarantee that the patient can give the best response, ensure that all assistive devices such as glasses and hearing aids are in place. Some older patients may need to limit the intensity rating to verbal descriptors, such as mild, moderate, or severe. Be sure to give the patient enough time to give as accurate a rating as possible. Most older patients can use a 0 to 10 scale if they are given enough time to respond.

- **Duration:** Ask the patient how long he or she has been in pain. Does the pain last all day? All night? Only when walking? If the patient replies that he or she has had the pain for years, ask when the pain began and whether something caused the pain to occur. Pain that has been present for a long time can be much more difficult to treat. For patients who have a memory impairment, a family member may be able to provide a good estimate of pain duration by reporting when the patient started to limp, change activity patterns, or have trouble sleeping.

- **Description:** This is an extremely important piece of the pain assessment. When the patient reports dull, achy pain, most often the source is musculoskeletal. However, when the patient reports burning, shooting, or tingling pain, the source may be neuropathic, which requires a different type of treatment.

- **Aggravating or alleviating factors:** Ask the patient what creates the pain and what makes the pain worse. Some older patients have their own special home remedies, such as topical creams and salves, which they use for almost everything. Encourage the older patient to share his or her techniques for pain control; frequently the patient is using heating pads or packs.

- **Functional impairment:** Pain is dynamic and increases with activity (Dahl & Kehlet, 2006). All patients can expect that activity will increase pain. For the older patient, this question may reveal an inability to do self-care. When this is the case, the patient may come to the clinic appointment looking unkempt or disheveled. As pain has an impact on their daily life, patients may retreat from increasing pain by staying in their homes or apartments. Social isolation can result—which, in turn, can cause depression and make the pain worse.

- **Cognitive impairment:** Cognitive impairment may be insidious. Patients may not realize they are losing cognitive function that can impair communication skills and perception. For each visit, it is important to perform a comprehensive assessment that includes evaluating any cognitive deficits.

- **Pain goal:** Try to set a reasonable pain level or intensity goal with the patient. Most older patients do not expect to be pain-free, but will have a certain level of pain they can tolerate to remain functional. Ask the patient to settle on a pain level that they feel is acceptable to them and will maximize their functionality with comfort. Target your pain management interventions to meet the pain goal that has been set.

(American Society for Pain Management Nursing, 2009; D'Arcy, 2007a, 2007b; Hadjistavropoulos et al., 2007)

Health care providers may never be able to discern why patients withhold pertinent information; however, they can use their observation skills to see if the patient is ambulating without hesitation, uses chair arms to get up from a sitting position, or appears sleep-deprived. Using these clues as part of the assessment process may uncover a hidden source of pain that, once treated, can significantly improve the older patient's quality of life.

> **Clinical Tip**
>
> For successful pain assessment, believe the patient's report of pain and respect the information shared with you. Creating an atmosphere of trust is critical to obtaining important information about a patient's pain.

ASSESSING ACUTE PAIN

Acute pain is pain that has a sudden onset. It may be the result of a fall or other injury. Older patients are more likely to treat this type of pain themselves or hope that it will go away. The delay in treatment may make the pain much more difficult to manage. Untreated acute pain can result in a chronic, centrally mediated pain condition such as complex regional pain syndrome (CRPS) that is much more difficult to treat (D'Arcy, 2007a).

Because of visual impairments, balance difficulties, and, in some cases, osteoporosis, older patients have the potential for more orthopedic injuries such as hip fractures, ankle strains and sprains, and wrist fractures. The prevalence of osteoarthritis in older patients also means that hip, shoulder, and knee replacements are much more common. Chronic illnesses such as diabetes, rheumatoid arthritis, and peripheral vascular disease can also cause significant pain (Bruckenthal & D'Arcy, 2007). Assessing pain in older patients with these conditions

> **Acute Pain**
>
> Acute pain is pain that is the result of tissue injury, trauma, or surgery. Its purpose is to warn the body that it has been injured. Acute pain is not expected to last long; its resolution is expected within the normal healing period (American Pain Society, 2009).

can be difficult because the hospital setting might be unfamiliar, and surgical medications might create sedation and confusion.

The Numeric Pain Rating (NRS) Scale

The best tool for assessing acute pain in the older patient who can self-report and has no or minimal cognitive impairments is the unidimensional Numeric Pain Rating (NRS) scale (see Figure 2.1).

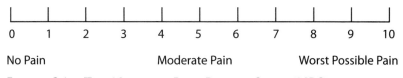

FIGURE 2.1   The Numeric Pain Rating Scale (NRS)

To perform a pain assessment using this tool, the patient is asked to rate his or her pain on a 0 to 10 Likert-type scale, where 0 equals no pain and 10 equals the worst pain possible. In a systematic review of 164 journal articles on pain, Jensen (2003) found that single-item ratings of pain intensity provided a reliable and valid measurement of pain intensity.

Clinical Tip

The NRS scale is the best scale to use when comparing pain ratings to determine if an intervention is effective or pain is decreasing. A decrease of two points or 30% on the NRS is considered to be significant (Gordon et al., 2002).

The Visual Analog Scale

The Visual Analog Scale is another unidimensional variation on the Likert scale (see Figure 2.2). Patients simply mark a line that corresponds with the amount of pain they are feeling. Patients with visual impairment can find this scale difficult to use, so some older patients might have difficulty marking the correct spot on the line (D'Arcy, 2003; Herr & Mobily, 1993).

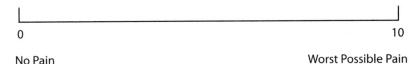

0   10

No Pain   Worst Possible Pain

FIGURE 2.2   THE VISUAL ANALOG SCALE

THE VERBAL DESCRIPTOR SCALE (VDS)

The Verbal Descriptor Scale, shown in Figure 2.3, uses a different approach and provides phrases such as "no pain," "moderate pain," or "worst possible pain" to help patients rate the intensity. Older patients with cognitive impairments will have difficulty using this scale if they do not understand the meaning of the words being used to rate the pain. In a study of cognitively impaired adult patients, Feldt, Ryden, and Miles (1998) found the participants were able to use this scale and had a 73% completion rate. In the clinical situation, some patients prefer to use words to describe their pain (D'Arcy, 2003; Herr & Mobily 1993).

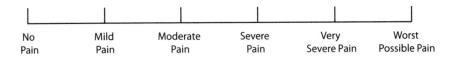

| No Pain | Mild Pain | Moderate Pain | Severe Pain | Very Severe Pain | Worst Possible Pain |

FIGURE 2.3   THE VERBAL DESCRIPTOR SCALE (VDS)

Clinical Tip

The words that patients use to describe their pain can be extremely important. If patients use terms such as burning, painful numbness, or tingling, the pain may be neuropathic and require different types of medications, such as gabapentin (Neurontin), to achieve adequate pain control.

THE COMBINED SCALE/THERMOMETER CONFIGURATION

The Thermometer Pain Scale uses numeric ratings and verbal descriptors to rate a patient's pain. This approach can allow the patient to choose the type of pain assessment that they feel works best.

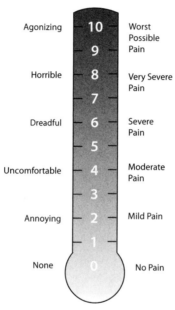

FIGURE 2.4   PAIN/DISTRESS INTENSITY SCALE

Clinical Tip

No matter what method is being used for pain assessment, the same tool should be used consistently. Documenting in the patient's record which tool is best suited for the patient and which tool is being used will allow for consistent pain assessment and make it possible to identify improvement in pain relief.

ASSESSING CHRONIC PAIN

Assessing chronic, persistent pain requires a more complex tool than assessing acute pain. Because chronic pain affects not only the patient's physical being but also his or her psychosocial and spiritual well-being, a more in-depth assessment of the pain is needed. The following multi-dimensional tools have been designed for this type of assessment:

- The McGill Pain Question-naire (MPQ)

- The Brief Pain Inventory (BPI)

- The Brief Pain Impact Questionnaire (BPIQ)

> **Clinical Tip**
>
> Chronic or persistent pain is pain that lasts beyond the normal healing period. It may be present even without evidence of damage on x-rays or scans. If pain lasts beyond 3 to 6 months, it is considered to be chronic.

These multidimensional tools share the following basic elements:

- Measurement of the pain's intensity, both current and past

- Description of the pain, using either a body diagram or words

- Measurement of the impact of the pain on daily activities, such as walking, sleeping, and so forth

Multidimensional assessment tools are longer and more complex than unidimensional tools. They require that the older patient be able to understand the words and descriptors and have the physical ability to complete the tool. Some of the tools can be administered either by the patient self-reporting pain, or by the nurse interviewing the patient. The latter option may provide a more accurate assessment.

The most current recommendation for assessing pain in older adults suggests the following:

- Include an assessment of all comorbid conditions that can affect pain.

- Assess for physical performance and balance using a tool such as the Physical Performance Test (PPT).

- Assess for perceived control over pain, depression, and anxiety using tools such as the Beck Anxiety Inventory, the Pain Anxiety Symptoms Scale, and the Geriatric Depression Scale.

- Combine the results of several different scales that represent various domains of the pain experience, so that a more complete picture of the pain experience for the older patient can be obtained.

  (Hadjistavropoulos et al., 2007)

THE McGILL PAIN QUESTIONNAIRE (MPQ)

The McGill Pain Questionnaire (MPQ) is one of the earlier tools for assessing pain. It has been translated into several different languages and is used in a variety of clinical settings, such as measuring post-procedural pain or experimentally induced pain, and in a large number of medical-surgical areas with a variety of patient populations.

The MPQ has both a short form and a long form, although the short form is more commonly used, because all the pertinent information for the pain assessment can be derived using it (see Figure 2.5). The MPQ has been determined to be reliable and valid to assess pain in patients, and it has been used both clinically and in research (Melzack, 1975, 1987).

The MPQ includes the following elements:

- A present pain intensity rating (PPI)

- A pain rating index

- Verbal descriptors that can be weighted and scored as indicators of the dimensions of the pain experience

  (Chok, 1998; Graham, Bond, Gerkovich, & Cook, 1980; McDonald & Weiskopf, 2001; McIntyre et al., 1995; Melzack, 1975, 1987; Wilkie, 1990)

Short-Form McGill Pain Questionnaire		(SF-MPQ)	Form X

A.   PLEASE DESCRIBE YOUR PAIN DURING THE LAST WEEK. *(Check off one box per line.)*

	None	Mild	Moderate	Severe
1. Throbbing	0 ☐	1 ☐	2 ☐	3 ☐
2. Shooting	0 ☐	1 ☐	2 ☐	3 ☐
3. Stabbing	0 ☐	1 ☐	2 ☐	3 ☐
4. Sharp	0 ☐	1 ☐	2 ☐	3 ☐
5. Cramping	0 ☐	1 ☐	2 ☐	3 ☐
6. Gnawing	0 ☐	1 ☐	2 ☐	3 ☐
7. Hot-Burning	0 ☐	1 ☐	2 ☐	3 ☐
8. Aching	0 ☐	1 ☐	2 ☐	3 ☐
9. Heavy (like a weight)	0 ☐	1 ☐	2 ☐	3 ☐
10. Tender	0 ☐	1 ☐	2 ☐	3 ☐
11. Splitting	0 ☐	1 ☐	2 ☐	3 ☐
12. Tiring-Exhausting	0 ☐	1 ☐	2 ☐	3 ☐
13. Sickening	0 ☐	1 ☐	2 ☐	3 ☐
14. Fear-Causing	0 ☐	1 ☐	2 ☐	3 ☐
15. Punishing-Cruel	0 ☐	1 ☐	2 ☐	3 ☐

B.   PLEASE RATE YOUR PAIN DURING THE LAST WEEK

The following line represents pain of increasing intensity from "no pain" to "worst possible pain".
Place a vertical mark (|) across the line in the position that best describes your pain **during the last week.**

| No Pain   Worst Possible Pain |

Score in mm
(Investigator's Use Only)

C.   CURRENT PAIN INTENSITY

0 ☐ No pain   3 ☐ Distressing
1 ☐ Mild   4 ☐ Horrible
2 ☐ Discomforting   5 ☐ Excruciating

Questionnaire developed by
Ronald Melzack

Copyright R. Melzack, 1987

FIGURE 2.5   THE MCGILL PAIN QUESTIONNAIRE (MPQ)—SHORT FORM

The most negative aspect of the MPQ is the use of a large number of verbal pain descriptors. For older patients this can be problematic, since the subtle variations to some of the terms and the severity ranking could be confusing. In the past, verbal descriptors selected by patients were determined to be more descriptive of syndromes rather than the individual pain complaint (Gracely, 1992; Graham et al., 1980).

THE BRIEF PAIN INVENTORY (BPI)

Another early multidimensional pain scale is the Brief Pain Inventory (BPI), originally designed to assess pain in patients with cancer (see Figure 2.6). It is a simple, easy-to-use instrument that studies have determined to be reliable and valid (Daut, Cleeland, & Flannery, 1983; Raiche, Osborne, Jensen, & Cardenas, 2006; Tan, Jensen, Thornby, & Shanti, 2004; Tittle, McMillan, & Hagan, 2003; Williams, Smith, & Fehnel, 2006). And, like the MPQ, the BPI has been translated into a number of languages and tested for reliability and validity (Ger, Ho, Sun, Wang, & Cleeland, 1999; Klepstad et al., 2002; Radbruch et al., 1999; Mystakidou et al., 2002).

One advantage of the BPI is the ability to use it either as a self-reporting instrument or during a patient interview. For older patients who may have difficulty filling out a paper form, being able to use the tool during an interview is advantageous.

The BPI includes the following components:

- A body diagram to mark the location of the pain

- A pain intensity rating

- A functional assessment to determine the impact of pain on daily activities

- Questions about pain medication efficacy

The successful use of the BPI requires the patient to have a relatively high level of understanding and fairly intact cognitive ability. If the patient is unable to provide the detailed information required by the tool, a different method of pain assessment might provide better results.

BRIEF PAIN INVENTORY

Date _____ / _____ / _____   Time:_____

Name: _____ _____ _____
        Last   First   Middle Initial

1) Throughout our lives, most of us have had pain from time to time (such as minor headaches, sprains, and toothaches). Have you had pain other than these everyday kinds of pain today?

   1. Yes   2. No

2) On the diagram, shade in the areas where you feel pain. Put an X on the area that hurts the most.

Right   Left   Left   Right

3) Please rate your pain by circling the one number that best describes your pain at its **WORST** in the last 24 hours.

0 1 2 3 4 5 6 7 8 9 10
No Pain   Pain as bad as you can imagine

4) Please rate your pain by circling the one number that best describes your pain at its **LEAST** in the last 24 hours.

0 1 2 3 4 5 6 7 8 9 10
No Pain   Pain as bad as you can imagine

5) Please rate your pain by circling the one number that best describes your pain on the **AVERAGE**.

0 1 2 3 4 5 6 7 8 9 10
No Pain   Pain as bad as you can imagine

6) Please rate your pain by circling the one number that tells how much pain you have **RIGHT NOW**.

0 1 2 3 4 5 6 7 8 9 10
No Pain   Pain as bad as you can imagine

7) What treatments or medications are you receiving for your pain?

_____

_____

8) In the last 24 hours, how much relief have pain treatments or medications provided? Please circle the one percentage that shows how much RELIEF you have received.

0% 10 20 30 40 50 60 70 80 90 100%
No Relief   Complete Relief

9) Circle the one number that describes how, during the past 24 hours, pain has interfered with your:

A) General activity

0 1 2 3 4 5 6 7 8 9 10
Does Not   Completely
Interfere   Interferes

B) Mood

0 1 2 3 4 5 6 7 8 9 10
Does Not   Completely
Interfere   Interferes

C) Walking ability

0 1 2 3 4 5 6 7 8 9 10
Does Not   Completely
Interfere   Interferes

D) Normal work (includes both work outside the home and housework)

0 1 2 3 4 5 6 7 8 9 10
Does Not   Completely
Interfere   Interferes

E) Relations with other people

0 1 2 3 4 5 6 7 8 9 10
Does Not   Completely
Interfere   Interferes

F) Sleep

0 1 2 3 4 5 6 7 8 9 10
Does Not   Completely
Interfere   Interferes

G) Enjoyment of life

0 1 2 3 4 5 6 7 8 9 10
Does Not   Completely
Interfere   Interferes

Copyright Charles Cleeland, 1991

FIGURE 2.6   BRIEF PAIN INVENTORY (BPI)

THE BRIEF PAIN IMPACT QUESTIONNAIRE

The Brief Pain Impact Questionnaire (BPIQ; see Figure 2.7) was developed as a quick, easy way to assess pain. Basically, it is a series of questions that provide information on pain intensity, functional impairment, health status, and alcohol use. Designed to be used during an interview, the BPIQ can help to pinpoint problem areas, such as functional impairment, very quickly.

BRIEF PAIN QUESTIONNAIRE*

- How strong is your pain, right now, worst/average over the past week?
- How many days over the past week have you been unable to do what you would like to do because of your pain?
- Over the past week, how often has pain interfered with your ability to take care of yourself, for example, with bathing, eating, dressing, and going to the toilet?
- Over the past week, how often has pain interfered with your ability to take care of your home-related chores such as grocery shopping, preparing meals, paying bills, and driving?
- How often do you participate in pleasurable activities such as hobbies, socializing with friends, and travel? Over the past week, how often has pain interfered with these activities?
- How often do you do some type of exercise? Over the past week, how often has pain interfered with your ability to exercise?
- Does pain interfere with your ability to think clearly?
- Does pain interfere with your appetite? Have you lost weight?
- Does pain interfere with your sleep? How often over the last week?
- Has pain interfered with your energy, mood, personality, or relationships with other people?
- Over the past week, have you taken pain medications?
- Has your use of alcohol or other drugs ever caused a problem for you or those close to you?
- How would you rate your health at the present time?

(Weiner, Herr, Rudy, 2002). *Used with permission of the author

---

FIGURE 2.7   BRIEF PAIN IMPACT QUESTIONNAIRE (BPQI)

PAIN ASSESSMENT IN NONVERBAL PATIENTS

Some of the patients most difficult to assess are those who cannot self-report pain. A number of tools can assess pain in this patient population. These tools, which are in earlier stages of development than the instruments previously described, primarily are based on the health care provider or caregiver's observations of the patient for behaviors that indicate pain. Recommendations for using a behavioral pain scale include

- Ask the patient to attempt to self-report his or her pain intensity.

- Try to identify any potential causes of pain, such as decubiti or undetected fractures.

- Take time to observe the patient, especially with movement, to detect previously unreported pain.

- Ask the family or other caregivers about the behaviors that indicate pain for the patient.

- Attempt an analgesic trial.

    (Hadjistavropoulos et al., 2007; Herr, Bjoro, & Decker et al., 2006)

One of the best references for behaviors that indicate pain is the Checklist of Nonverbal Pain Indicators (CNPI). It is a list of six behaviors that have been determined to indicate the presence of pain (Feldt, 2000; Feldt, Ryden & Miles, 1998). To determine which behaviors indicate pain, a study was conducted comparing cognitively impaired to noncognitively impaired patients with a similar source of pain (Feldt). The checklist was designed for use with older cognitively impaired adults in acute care settings (Herr, Bjoro, & Decker et al., 2006). The following behaviors were identified:

- Vocalizations

- Facial grimacing

- Bracing

- Rubbing

- Restlessness

- Vocal complaints, such as moaning

Building on this concept, the American Geriatrics Society's 2002 guideline for treating persistent pain in older adults identified the following behaviors as indicating pain:

- Verbalizations, such as moaning, calling out, asking for help, and groaning

- Facial expressions, such as grimacing, frowning, wrinkling the forehead, and other distorted expressions

- Body movements, such as rigid and tense body posture, guarding, rocking, fidgeting, pacing, and massaging the painful area

- Changes in interpersonal interactions, such as aggression, combative behavior, resisting care, and being disruptive or withdrawn

- Changes in mental status, such as crying, increased confusion, irritability, or distress

  (AGS, 2002)

Clinical Tip

It may not be possible to assign a numeric equivalent for pain using a behavioral pain scale (Herr, Bjoro, & Decker et al., 2006). However, with a scale that is set up for a numeric rating of pain, the numeric range can be used as a trigger to treat pain. For example, a behavioral scale pain rating of 4 to 6 would be best treated with a moderate-level pain medication. When pain is suspected, a trial of pain medication can help determine the presence of pain if pain behaviors lessen.

A variety of pain scales assess pain in the nonverbal older patient population. What these tools have in common is the use of a set of behavior categories, such as restlessness and body tension, to assess the patient for the presence of pain. Although it is easy to say that a patient with a hip fracture is in pain, providing a tool that has consistent assessment criteria can help standardize the assessment process and drive care. Two tools currently used to assess pain in nonverbal patient populations are the modified Faces, Legs, Activity, Cry, Consolability (FLACC) scale and the Pain Assessment in Advanced Dementia (PAINAD) scale.

THE MODIFIED FLACC SCALE

The modified FLACC scale (see Figure 2.8) has been adapted for adults from the pediatric format and can be used for nonverbal patients in any setting. It consists of behavioral elements such as facial expression, body rigidity, and restlessness. Each of the five behavior categories is ranked as behavior absent (0), behavior present (1), or behavior very prevalent (2). For example, the body rigidity/tension section might be scored as follows:

- 0 - Body relaxed
- 1 - Intermittent tension
- 2 - Body rigid

In this scale, the behavioral ratings can be converted to a numeric equivalent. It is important to consider that the conversion process is imprecise at best. However, finding a range for the severity of the behaviors can provide some insight into the pain experience of patients and help drive a treatment plan to address the pain. Training nurses to monitor a patient for specific pain behaviors by using a scale can help ensure that patients who have pain and cannot communicate are not being overlooked.

BEHAVIORAL PAIN SCALE (NONVERBAL) FOR PATIENTS UNABLE TO PROVIDE A SELF-REPORT OF PAIN				
FACE	**0** Face muscles relaxed	**1** Facial muscle tension, frown, grimace	**2** Frequent to constant frown, clenched jaw	**Face Score:**
RESTLESSNESS	**0** Quite relaxed appearance, normal movement	**1** Occasional restless movement, shifting position	**2** Frequent restless movement may include extremities or head	**Restlessness Score:**
MUSCLE TONE*	**0** Normal muscle tone, relaxed	**1** Increased tone, flexion of fingers and toes	**2** Rigid tone	**Muscle Tone Score:**
VOCALIZATION**	**0** No abnormal sounds	**1** Occasional moans, cries, whimpers, or grunts	**2** Frequent or continuous moans, cries, whimpers, or grunts	**Vocalization Score:**
CONSOLABILITY	**0** Content, relaxed	**1** Reassured by touch or talk. Distractible	**2** Difficult to comfort by touch or talk	**Consolability Score:**
Behavioral Pain Assessment Scale Total (0 – 10)				

Developed by Margaret Campbell, Detroit Receiving Hospital

*Assess muscle tone in patients with spinal cord lesion or injury at a level above the lesion or injury. Assess patients with hemiplegia on the unaffected side.

** This item cannot be measured in patients with artificial airways.

How to Use the Pain Assessment Behavioral Scale:

1. Observe behaviors and mark appropriate number for each category.

2. Total the numbers in the Pain Assessment Behavioral Score column.

3. No evidence of pain = zero. Mild pain = 1-3. Moderate pain = 4-6. Severe uncontrolled pain = > 6.

Considerations:

1. Use the standard pain scale whenever possible to obtain the patient's self-report of pain. Self-report is the best indicator of the presence and intensity of pain.

2. Use this scale for patients who are unable to provide a self-report of pain.

3. In addition, a "Proxy pain evaluation" from family, friends, or clinicians close to the patient may be helpful to evaluate pain based on previous knowledge of patient response.

4. When in doubt, provide an analgesic. "If there is reason to suspect pain, an analgesic trial can be diagnostic as well as therapeutic."

FIGURE 2.8   THE MODIFIED FLACC SCALE

THE PAINAD SCALE

Patients with dementia are at high risk for having pain that is not assessed or treated. One tool that has been found to be clinically appli-
cable is the PAINAD scale (see Figure 2.9).

	0	1	2	Score
Breathing	Normal	Occasional labored breathing Short period of hyperventilation	Noisy labored breathing Long period of hyperventilation Cheyne-stokes respirations	
Negative Vocalization	None	Occasional moan/ groan Low level speech/ negative or dis-approving quality	Repeated, troubled, calling out Loud moaning or groaning Crying	
Facial Expression	Smiling	Sad Frightened Frown	Facial grimacing inexpressive	
Body Language	Relaxed	Tense Distressed Pacing Fidgeting	Rigid Fists clenched Knees pulled up Pulling or pushing away Striking out	
Consolability	No need to console	Distracted or reassured by voice or touch	Unable to console, distract, or reassure	
				Total _____

Developed at the New England Geriatric Research Education and Clinical Center, EN Rogers Memorial Veter-
ans Hospital, Bedford MA.
Warden, V., Hurley, A.C., & Volicer, L. (2003). Development and psychometric evaluation of the Pain Assessment
in Advanced Dementia (PAINAD)Scale. *Journal of the American Medical Directors Association, 4,* 9-15.

FIGURE 2.9   THE PAINAD SCALE

The PAINAD scale, designed specifically for patients with dementia
or Alzheimer's disease who cannot self-report pain (Lane et al., 2003),
consists of the following five categories:

- Breathing

- Negative vocalizations

- Facial expression

- Body language

- Consolability

Each of the categories is rated as follows:

- 0 - Normal

- 1 - Occasionally present or present to a lesser degree

- 2 - Significant behavior such as unable to be consoled, repeated calling out, hyperventilation.

These ratings are then converted to a 0 to 10 pain intensity rating.

As with any behavioral scale, the ratings of the PAINAD scale rely on caregiver observations, which are not seen as totally accurate (Herr, 2006). Because the tool isolates only five behaviors, it is not considered comprehensive enough to ensure an accurate pain rating in patients with complex pain needs (Herr, 2006).

Additional Assessment Tools

In addition to the tools already mentioned, other tools can be effective for assessing the pain of older patients. For example, the Pain Assessment Checklist for Seniors with Limited Ability to Communicate (PACSLAC), the Functional Pain Scale (FPS), and the Doloplus-2 all show promise (Hadjistavropoulos et al., 2007).

SUMMARY

There is no doubt that pain assessment in older patients can be challenging and requires special techniques and tools. Nurses who care for these patients understand the need to have good, consistent assessments so that pain can be treated adequately. If pain is not assessed, it cannot be treated. Techniques such as around-the-clock dosing of pain medications, careful use of opioids and coanalgesic medications, and complementary therapies can be used to treat pain once it is assessed. Using reliable and valid pain assessment tools facilitates the adequate treatment of pain in older patients, to ensure the highest quality of life possible.

CASE STUDY

Mary Jones, 76, has just been transferred from her independent living facility to a skilled nursing facility. Mary had long ago said that she never wanted to live in a nursing home, but her condition has deteriorated to the point that skilled care is necessary.

Mary has had insulin-dependent diabetes for many years and has osteoarthritis in her knees. At her independent living facility, she had enjoyed the garden and card clubs. More recently, she had been staying in her room and was very irritable. She slept most of the day and found it difficult to cook and clean her apartment.

As Mary's nurse, you are assigned to do her admission assessment. When you go into her room, she seems sad and withdrawn. When you ask about her pain, Mary looks at you and says, "I hate the pain. It is always there. My feet burn and it hurts to walk. It's not enough that my knees are so achy, especially when the weather changes, but my feet are really the worst. I can't sleep at night, and putting on shoes is very hard to tolerate. If I could just have managed the pain, I could have stayed in my home. They ask me to rate my pain and I always tell them 6, but nothing ever helps." When you review Mary's medication sheets, you see that she has an order to take 350 mg of acetaminophen every 6 hours or as needed, although none has been taken in the past 24 hours.

Critical Analysis Questions

1. Use the basic elements of assessment to assess Mary's pain.

2. How impaired is her functional status, and what impact has it had on her quality of life?

3. What would be a reasonable pain goal for Mary?

4. How would you include the pain assessment process in Mary's plan of care?

5. What could the potential outcome be for Mary if her pain was assessed regularly and a suitable treatment prescribed and administered?

3

PAIN MEDICATION MANAGEMENT FOR OLDER ADULTS

Pain medication management for patients older than 65 years of age can be very challenging. As mentioned in Chapter 1, many myths can lead to undertreated and undermanaged pain in that population. Older patients are not included in many clinical trials, so determining drug choices, dosing limits, and side-effect profiles is, in the main, subjective. In a report of 83 randomized trials for nonsteroidal anti-inflammatory drugs (NSAIDs), with 10,000 subjects, only 2.3% of the participants were more than 65 years old, and none was older than 85 (American Geriatrics Society [AGS], 2002). Also, health care professionals are afraid to prescribe opioid medication because they are afraid of adverse side effects—such as sedation, nausea, or constipation—that can occur with these medications.

The following myths help explain why managing pain medication in this population is challenging:

For prescribers:

- The notion that older patients cannot tolerate opioid medications

- The notion that older patients do not experience pain in the same way that younger patients do

For patients:

- The notion that older patients expect pain to be a part of their daily lives

- The notion that older patients want to be seen as good patients who do not make trouble for others
  (Karani & Meier, 2004)

Older patients *do* have more comorbidities than younger patients, which makes prescribing pain medication more complex. But, the preceding myths can lead to significant pain and depression when health care providers offer them less effective medication or tell them that they must learn to live with chronic pain. The issue is not so much that older patients cannot tolerate pain medications, but rather is more a function of

- How age has affected their physiology, such as liver and kidney functions that clear medications of all types

- Their attitudes toward pain and using pain medications in general

Reluctance to take pain medication, for whatever reason, may play a significant role in unresolved pain. Most older patients do not like to take medication for anything, including pain. They may take it as prescribed, take it as they feel they need it, or not take it at all if the side effects are too problematic. They fully understand the need for medications, but they wish to have more control over how they take the medication.

One in five older patients reported taking pain medication only occasionally during a 1-week period of time (Reyes-Gibby, Aday, Todd, Cleeland, & Anderson, 2007). This finding may be the result of

- Undertreatment by prescribers
- Inability to afford the high cost of medications
- Reluctance to take pain medication
- Fear that reporting pain might create the need for expensive tests or hospitalization

  (Reyes-Gibby, Aday, Todd, Cleeland, & Anderson, 2007)

For older patients, these misperceptions lead directly to untreated and undertreated pain that has significant consequences, including

- Depression
- Impaired cognition
- Sleep disturbances
- Poorer clinical outcomes
- Decreased functional ability
- Decreased quality of life
- Anxiety
- Decreased socialization
- Increased health care utilization and costs

  (AGS, 2009; D'Arcy, 2007; Karani & Meier, 2004)

PAIN MEDICATION USE IN OLDER PATIENTS

Older patients can experience a pain stimulus in the same way younger patients can (Huffman & Kunik, 2000; McLennon, 2005). However, the nervous systems of older patients are more likely to have altered neural transmission related to chronic diseases such as diabetes, neuropathies, or arthritis. Not only can pain be transmitted differently, but how a patient's body uses medications also may change as the body ages. Selecting a medication that relieves pain, but does not produce adverse side effects or interfere with any other medication the patient is taking, can be very difficult when the patient is older.

> ### Clinical Tip
> Physiologic changes resulting from aging vary among older adults; no two patients are the same, nor do they age the same.

Naturally, the older patient comes to the experience of using pain medications with an older body. Some of the more significant changes that affect the use of opioid medications involve organ systems:

- Kidney mass decreases 25%-30% between the ages of 30 and 80. The resulting decreased renal function can affect drug excretion, so dosing adjustments must be made when prescribing medications that are excreted renally.

- Increases in mu opioid receptors, coupled with a slowed gastrointestinal (GI) motility, can easily increase constipation.

- Vascular changes are common in older patients, producing orthostatic hypotension, fluid retention, dizziness, and an increased potential for falls.

- After age 65 patients can expect a decline in visual acuity, and after age 75, an additional decline in depth perception. Hearing loss can affect 25%-45% of patients older than 65 years of age. This can affect how patients see the medication instructions and hear the directions for taking them.

(Adapted from Potter, 2004)

Other reasons why older patients have difficulty using medication and experience adverse effects include

- Body fat composition: Muscle-to-fat ratio changes as patients age.

- Protein binding affects drug effectiveness. Poor nutrition can decrease protein stores and affect the protein binding capacity of certain medications. Thus, drugs might compete for protein binding sites, rendering one or more of the medications ineffective.

- Age affects functions that impact the absorption, metabolism, and clearance of medications, including a slowed GI motility, decreased cardiac output, and decreased glomerular filtration rate.

- Changes in sensory and cognitive perception, such as sedation or confusion, may be a risk for some patients, due to potential side effects of both nonopioid and opioid medications such as antidepressants and anticonvulsants.

- Drug excretion and elimination are reduced by 10% for each decade after the age of 40, because of decreased renal function.

(Bruckenthal & D'Arcy, 2007; Horgas, 2003)

Special Considerations with Medication Use

For patients who are nonverbal and unable to communicate, asking for pain medications when pain is present is not an option. For these patients, using a trial of pain medication when pain is suspected provides an indication if pain is the actual problem. If pain is present, patients may have an increase in their usual pain behaviors and a disruption in rest or activities.

To effectively treat pain in this population, using an around-the-clock medication regimen rather than an as-needed dosing schedule will provide more consistent pain relief. If the patient becomes too sedated with this approach, holding the medication and changing the schedule or dose may provide better pain relief without side effects.

Polypharmacy

Given that older patients have many more comorbidities, polypharmacy, the use of more than five prescribed medications per day, is common. Not only will the older patient be using the prescribed medications, but there also may be outdated prescription medications being mixed into the medication regimen or over-the-counter medications being used regularly. The potential for drug-drug interaction and side effects is increased with this use pattern.

Polypharmacy should be avoided, if possible, in the older adult. However, multidrug therapy is a reality for many older patients with multiple comorbidities. Even if the definition of polypharmacy is expanded to nine medications, as has been suggested, most older patients would still fall into this category (Zurakowski, 2009).

Zurakowski (2009) suggests that prescribers follow what has been described as "rational polypharmacy," in which the Beers criteria, a list of medications that may cause side effects in the elderly, and the pharmacist help to determine safer combinations of medications for patients. Drug-drug interactions can cause serious side effects that should be avoided. Prescribers should check the current medication list against the medication they are considering prescribing, to make sure there is no potential for drug-drug interactions.

Polypharmacy

Polypharmacy is defined as five or more prescribed medications. The average older adult has 6.5 chronic conditions, commonly resulting in multidrug therapy (Zurakowski, 2009).

Most patients tend to keep medications they are no longer using, in case they would have a similar complaint. Older patients are no different, but they may have a more extensive collection because of their age. Medications that are outdated or no longer being used should be discarded. Patients should have a current medication list that health care providers can use to determine which medications are current and what doses are being used. Nursing home residents should have a current medication list sent with them when they are transferred to a hospital for acute care.

For primary care patients, the health care provider should ask the patient/family to bring all medications that the patient is taking. These "brown bag" sessions can uncover a variety of outdated medications from multiple prescribers who are not aware of the medications being prescribed by second or third health care providers (D'Arcy, 2007). After the current medication list is updated, the medications should be checked for potential drug-drug interactions. If drug-drug interactions are discovered, the health care provider should be notified and the medications changed to those that do not interact. For patient safety, older patients can benefit from periodic checks of medication bottles, pill checks, and brown bag sessions to ensure that the medications are being taken as prescribed, and that there are no adverse effects. In addition to patient education, patients should be given information regarding whom to call with questions or concerns about medication.

PAIN MEDICATION MANAGEMENT FOR NONVERBAL PATIENTS

Providing pain medication for demented, cognitively impaired, or non-communicative patients can present another challenge. Although these patients may have not felt pain differently, they may have trouble interpreting the sensation as pain, depending on the amount of neuronal loss (McLennon, 2005). Many of these patients are long-term care residents, but there is also a cohort who is being cared for at home. For the patient who has family available, getting information on the patient's usual pain behaviors and effective treatments can help when developing a plan of care.

The prevalence of pain in demented individuals is not known (Horgas, 2003). Since these patients are in varying stages of their disease, their ability to report pain is also wide-ranging. Using an observational behavioral pain measure (see "The PAINAD Scale" in Chapter 2) can help to determine if the patient is experiencing pain and aid in decisions about medication choices. Given the difficulties in recognizing pain in this population, it is not hard to understand the problem of getting adequate treatment for pain.

In a study of nursing home residents, impaired residents were prescribed and administered significantly less analgesic medication than were intact residents (Horgas, 2003). In another study, demented patients with hip fractures were given three times less analgesic medication than nonimpaired patients with similar conditions (Horgas).

The following are recommendations for treating pain in nonverbal patients:

- Make an observational assessment, noting behaviors—such as grimacing—that indicate pain.

- Conduct a clinical trial of pain medications to see if pain behaviors decrease.

- Use nonpharmacologic pain-management strategies, as well as medications.
  (Horgas, 2003)

Regardless of the approach, patients who cannot self-report pain or ask for pain medication must have access to pain relief measures, including medication. If a trial of pain medication produces reduced pain behaviors or otherwise seems to be effective, administering the medication around the clock can provide significant relief and improve quality of life for nonverbal patients (McLennon, 2005).

CHOOSING THE RIGHT PAIN MEDICATION

The World Health Organization (WHO) "ladder" provides a good method for determining which medication fits a pain complaint (see Figure 3.1).

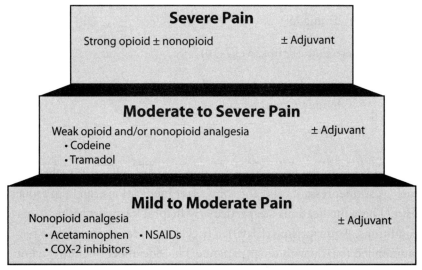

Severe Pain
Strong opioid ± nonopioid   ± Adjuvant

Moderate to Severe Pain
Weak opioid and/or nonopioid analgesia   ± Adjuvant
• Codeine
• Tramadol

Mild to Moderate Pain
Nonopioid analgesia   ± Adjuvant
• Acetaminophen   • NSAIDs
• COX-2 inhibitors

COX=cyclooxygena se; NSAIDs=nonsteroidal anti-inflammatory drugs.
Berry, P.H., Covington, E.C., Dahl, J.L., Katz, J.A., & Mia Skowski, C. (2006). Pain: Current understanding of assessment, management, and treatments. Reston, VA: National Pharmaceutical Council, Inc., and Joint Commission on Accreditation of Healthcare Organizations.

FIGURE 3.1   WORLD HEALTH ORGANIZATION PAIN "LADDER"

Originally developed for use with cancer patients, the ladder uses the following approach to choosing a pain medication:

1. Mild Pain (Pain Level 1-3)

   • Acetaminophen

   • NSAIDs (both nonselective and COX-2 selective)

2. Moderate Pain (Pain Level 4-6)

- Combination medications: acetaminophen and oxycodone, codeine, or hydrocodone

- Oxycodone (short-acting or extended release)

- Oxymorphone (short-acting or extended release)

- Tramadol

3. Severe Pain (Pain Level 7-10)

- Opioid medications such as morphine, hydromorphone, fentanyl, methadone

(Dalton & Youngblood, 2001; D'Arcy, 2007)

In addition to the primary medication for pain, adjuvant medications such as antidepressants and anticonvulsant medications can help reduce pain. These medications are particularly helpful for neuropathic pain conditions. Amitriptyline (Elavil), a tricyclic antidepressant, is not recommended for use with older patients. The side effect of amitriptyline that is most concerning for the older patient is morning orthostatic hypotension, which increases the risk for falls.

The idea of starting low and going slow when using opioid medications for pain is a good approach. Trialing small doses of opioids and having the family observe the patient for any changes in clarity can be very helpful in determining the best opioid to use for pain relief.

PAIN MEDICATIONS FOR MILD PAIN

When patients are having mild pain, they may tend to use an over-the-counter medication, which can include acetaminophen or an NSAID compound. Although these medications are readily available, they are not without risks.

Acetaminophen

Acetaminophen is available as an over-the-counter medication in a variety of formulas and strengths. Acetaminophen is valuable for treating mild pain and can be used as an adjunct medication to opioids. Once pain reaches higher levels, most patients consider acetaminophen to have little value; however, when used in combination with opioids, acetaminophen can decrease pain and help reduce the dose of opioid drugs.

The total daily dose of acetaminophen should be decreased if there is liver impairment. If the patient has a history of alcohol abuse, or liver or renal impairment, the maximum daily dose of acetaminophen, 4 g per day, should be decreased by 50% to 75%, or it should not used at all (AGS, 2009).

Clinical Tip

Because acetaminophen is metabolized in the liver, monitor liver function tests (LFTs) at least annually for patients who are taking acetaminophen regularly. There have been cases of transient elevations of alanine amino-tranferase with patients using acetaminophen long-term, but these have not been translated into liver failure or hepatic dysfunction if maximum doses are avoided (AGS, 2009).

NSAIDS

Nonsteroidal anti-inflammatory drugs (NSAIDs) have long been a standard for pain relief in older patients. Relatively cheap, they are easily accessible at most supermarkets or drugstores. They are available as over-the-counter formulations and in prescription strength. When used appropriately, NSAIDS are more effective in relieving chronic inflammatory pain than acetaminophen (AGS, 2009). The most common uses for NSAIDs are inflammatory pain, arthritis pain, headaches, and minor sprains and strains.

There are two basic classes of NSAIDs:

- **Nonselective NSAIDS:** The nonselective NSAIDS, such as ibuprofen (Motrin, Advil), naproxen (Naprosyn), and ketoprofen (Orudis), affect the production of the prostaglandins that coat and protect the lining of the stomach, as well as the prostaglandins found in other organs, such as the kidneys and the heart.

- **COX-2 selective NSAIDs:** The only COX-2 medication available at this time is Celebrex, which spares the stomach prostaglandins and does not affect platelet aggregation, so blood clotting is not affected.

Research from the Food and Drug Administration (FDA) indicates that all NSAIDs, not only the COX-2 selective medications such as Celebrex, have the potential for increased cardiovascular risk, renovascular risk, stroke, and myocardial infarction (Bennett, 2005; D'Arcy, 2007). GI bleeding also continues to be a risk with NSAIDs, and for those patients who are taking aspirin as a cardiac prophylaxis, the risk increases severalfold with concomitant NSAID and aspirin use (D'Arcy, 2007). A recent study reviewing hospital admission statistics indicates that in adults over the age of 65, NSAIDs were implicated in 23.5% of the GI bleeding cases (AGS, 2009).

> **For More Information**
>
> Mechanisms for both types of NSAIDs can be found at http://www.fda.gov/ohrms/dockets/ac/05/slides/2005-4090S1_02_FDA-Cryer.ppt.

Gastrointestinal Risks With NSAIDs

One of the major risks with nonselective NSAIDs is gastric ulceration. Gastric ulcers develop within a week in approximately 30% of patients started on nonselective NSAIDs (Wallace & Staats, 2005). Most patients with these ulcers are asymptomatic and seek medical care only when the bleeding becomes obvious with tarry stools or hematemesis.

To lessen the risk of GI bleeding, some practitioners commonly use a proton pump inhibitor (PPI) such as omeprazole (Prilosec), which provides protection only for the upper GI system. Adherence of patients taking a PPI for protection is suspect. A recent study found that by the time patients received three prescriptions for a PPI as a NSAID prophylaxis, the nonadherence rate was high, at 60.8% (Sturkenboom, Burke, Tangelder, Dieleman, & Walton et al., 2003).

Because many older patients are also taking aspirin daily for cardioprotective effect, adding the incidence of ulcer formation with aspirin to the NSAID risk only increases the potential for GI bleeding (AGS, 2009). Higher doses and older age are associated with a higher incidence of GI side effects (Perez-Gutthann, Rodriguez, & Raifoed, 1997). Additionally, chronic alcohol use with NSAIDs increases the risk for GI bleeding and ulceration. Whether GI issues are a consideration depends largely on the individual patient's history and medical situation.

Cardiovascular Risks With NSAIDs

There are certain patient groups who are at higher risk for cardiovascular events and for whom NSAIDs are not recommended, including patients who recently have had heart bypass surgery, patients with heart disease, and patients who have had transient ischemic attacks (TIAs) or strokes. For these patients, an alternate form of analgesic is recommended.

When trying to determine which NSAID to offer a patient, consider that there are indications that naproxen interferes with the inhibitory effect of aspirin (Capone, Sciulli, Tacconelli, Grana, & Ricciotti et al., 2005), and the same effect may be seen with concomitant use of ibuprofen, acetaminophen, and diclofenac (Catella-Lawson, Reilly, Kapoor, Cuicchiara, & DeMarco et al., 2001). Patients who take aspirin as a prophylaxis suffer an increased risk for GI events, and using NSAIDs may decrease the effectiveness of the aspirin.

In general, the recommendations for using NSAIDs for pain relief indicate that the medication should be used at the lowest dose for the shortest period of time (AHA, 2005). Older patients should be aware that continuing to take NSAIDs over the long term for arthritis or other chronic conditions could cause serious, life-threatening effects.

Opioid Use in Older Patients

Opioids are primarily mu agonist drugs, although they bind to three different types of receptors. Mu binding sites are found throughout the peripheral and central nervous system, the gastrointestinal system, and other locations. Kappa and delta binding sites are located in other areas of the body, such as the spinal cord, and are not as common as mu sites.

Analgesia results when the medication enters the body and finds the mu site, binds, and blocks the progression of the pain stimulus. The opioid binding sites in the bowel, along with slowed gastric emptying, contribute to the higher incidence of opioid-induced constipation in older patients (Zurakowski, 2009). Opioid binding sites are also located in the periphery, though the mechanism of action is still under discussion.

The initial goal of opioid administration is to produce analgesia with the least number of adverse effects. However, some elements of opioid therapy are beyond the control of the prescriber. The following factors can influence opioid metabolism and potentially affect analgesia:

- **Opioid polymorphism:** Opioid polymorphism relates to the ability of the medication to bind to a certain genetic variation of the binding site. For example, some patients may have mu binding sites that are genetically designed to more readily accept morphine than fentanyl. If given the nonpreferred drug, the patient may experience decreased pain relief (D'Arcy, 2007).

- **Binding ability:** Older patients may have a protein deficiency that decreases the binding ability of the drug (Bruckenthal & D'Arcy, 2007; Zurakowski, 2009).

- **The cytochrome P450 (CYP450) system in the liver:** This system transforms some opioids into usable metabolites (Fine & Portnoy, 2007).

- **The rate at which opioids are metabolized:** Metabolism of opioids may be poor, intermediate, extensive, or ultrarapid (Løvlie, Daly, Matre, Molven, & Steen, 2001).

- **Ethnic differences:** 5% to 10% of Caucasian patients are unable or have poor ability to metabolize codeine to morphine, the active metabolite (Løvlie et al., 2001).

Another important element to consider is the past history of the patient when opioids have been used. Were there any serious adverse effects with certain opioids? Did the patient's pain respond better to one particular opioid? Moreover, one of the most important aspects of using opioids with older patients is whether the patient actually continued to take the medication when it was last prescribed. If the older patient has had success with a particular opioid, it is worth trying to use that medication again for pain.

Opioid Terms

- Opioid naïve: A patient who has not been taking opioids prior to the start of opioid therapy.
- Opioid tolerant or dependent: A patient who takes opioid medications regularly (every day).

Using opioids in these two groups of patients is very different. Opioid-tolerant patients may require more medication for new pain, such as post-surgery pain. Opioid-naïve patients require more monitoring for adverse effects at the beginning of opioid therapy (D'Arcy, 2007).

When opioids are being started, the nurse should ask the patient whether he or she is using alcohol to help control pain. If medication does not decrease pain to an acceptable level, some patients might supplement the medication with alcohol to enhance its effect. This practice is very dangerous, and the nurse should be careful and nonjudgmental in approaching the topic. If the patient is using alcohol for adjunct pain relief, the nurse can help the patient communicate his or her need to the health care provider for better pain management that would not include the use of alcohol.

Opioids and Addiction

Older patients are also concerned about addiction. They may have had a friend or family member who had difficulty controlling opioid use, and they are likely aware of the public personalities who are reported in the news and on television as being addicted to their pain medications. Nurses who address this question can assure patients that addiction occurs very rarely in older patients (McLennon, 2005). Defining the meaning of addiction, dependence, tolerance, and pseudo-addiction is also helpful, so that the patient understands the difference. Because addiction rates among older patients are very low, it is a safe assumption that those who did not experience addiction in the past will have little or no problem using opioids for pain.

If the older patient has a history of addiction or substance abuse, you can still effectively treat pain, although higher doses will be needed.

For More Information

Addiction

Addiction is a chronic, neurobiologic disease characterized by the four C's:

- Craving for the substance
- Compulsive use
- Lack of control over substance use
- Continued use despite harm

    (American Pain Society [APS], ASAM, AAPM, 2001)

Physical Dependence

When patients take opioids on a daily basis to relieve pain, their bodies become dependent on receiving the medication regularly. If the patient stops taking the opioid, a withdrawal syndrome will occur. This syndrome is characterized by nausea, vomiting, diarrhea, shaking, and elevated blood pressure (AAPM, APS, ASAM, 2001).

Tolerance

Over time, the body can develop a tolerance, or lessening of the effects, of opioids—whether sedation, nausea, or pain relief. Patients who are experiencing tolerance may need to have their dosage increased (Warltier et al., 2004). Patients who experience tolerance are not becoming addicted to the medication; rather, they are showing physiologic accommodation over time (Jage & Bey, 2000).

Pseudo-Addiction

A set of behaviors such as clock watching or perceived drug seeking that are really an indication of undertreated pain. Once pain medication is adjusted, these behaviors disappear (Fine & Portnoy, 2007).

Opioids for Moderate Pain

The majority of the opioid medications for moderate pain are combination medications. These combinations of opioids with acetaminophen have a ceiling: The maximum daily dose of acetaminophen (Tylenol) is the limiting factor. The following medications are useful for treating moderate-level pain:

- **Codeine with or without acetaminophen (Tylenol #3):** Used for mild pain relief. Constipation and GI side effects are common.

- **Hydrocodone/APAP (Vicodin/Lortab, Lortab elixir, extended release Vicodin):** Usually well tolerated by patients. Has an extended release form. Elixir can be used for patients who have difficulty swallowing or have feeding tubes.

- **Oxycodone/APAP (Percocet, Percodan, Oxyfast, Oxycontin):** Provides high-grade pain relief and is commonly used for postoperative pain. Oxyfast elixir is well-tolerated. Oxycontin is the extended release form.

- **Oxymorphone (Opana, Opana ER):** Provides extended pain relief even with the immediate release form (Adams et al., 2005; Adams & Abdieh, 2004). Very little breakthrough medication is required with the extended release form. It is available in an IV form called Numorphan.

- **Tramadol (Ultram, Ultracet, Ultram ER):** A medication including a mu agonist and a selective serotonin reuptake inhibitor (SSRI). It lowers the seizure threshold but also has side effects of dizziness, constipation, nausea, and somnolence, making it difficult to use with older patients.

  (D'Arcy, 2007; APS, 2009)

Opioids for Severe Pain

When older patients have severe pain, it is difficult to start low and go slow, which is the recommended approach to treating pain in older patients. Using smaller amounts of opioids and adjusting the interval while monitoring for side effects can help to determine what amount of these potent, pure opioid medications will be most effective for pain relief, yet cause the fewest side effects.

- **Morphine (Morphine IR, MS Contin, Kadian, Avinza, Roxanol):** Morphine has a high profile for constipation, nausea, pruritis, and hallucinations. The elixir Roxanol is commonly used for oncology patients, or patients who cannot swallow or have feeding tubes. It is a very effective medication for pain relief, but the significant number of side effects may make it difficult for older patients to tolerate this medication.

- **Hydromorphone (Dilaudid):** Hydromorphone is a very potent pain medication—0.2 mg of intravenous hydromorphone is equal to 1 mg of intravenous morphine. Because of its potency, very small amounts of the drug can provide pain relief, yet reduce the potential for side effects.

- **Fentanyl (Duragesic patches, Fentora, Fentanyl Oralets):** Fentanyl is a medication that has no oral route for tablets, since it degrades in the gastric secretions. It is used as a transdermal patch or buccal preparations such as the Oralet and Fentora tablets. The Duragesic patch has a 12.5 mcg fentanyl per hour strength that can be useful for older patients who need around-the-clock pain relief and are opioid-tolerant. Buccal fentanyl should not be used in opioid naïve patients, since the preparations have a very rapid onset, while the patch can take anywhere from 12 to 18 hours for onset of action, with up to 48 hours to achieve a steady state.

- **Methadone (Dolophine):** Only very experienced prescribers should prescribe methodone (APS, 2009; Chou et al., 2009). The primary issue with methadone is its long half-life. The medication has a pain relief potential of 6 to 8 hours, while the medication half-life can extend to 12 to 150 hours, depending on the patient (Fine & Portnoy, 2007). Using methadone in an older patient requires an in-depth knowledge of the patient and medication. Once the drug is chosen, the therapy should be initiated at very small doses and monitored for side effects.

(Adapted from D'Arcy, 2007)

Opioids to Avoid

Over time, some pain medications have fallen out of favor because of toxic metabolites, side effects, and dosing concerns related to acetaminophen in combination medications. The two most commonly used medications that fall into this category are meperidine-pethadine, and propoxyphene.

- **Meperidine (pethidine, Demerol):** Meperidine should not be used, particularly in patients who have decreased renal clearance or kidney disease (APS, 2009; Fine & Portnoy, 2007). Additionally, the medication has a renally cleared metabolite, normeperidine, which can build up in the central nervous system and cause seizures (APS).

- **Propxyphene (Darvon, Darvocet):** A number of propoxyphene medications are also problematic for patients, particularly older patients. The medications should be considered for mild pain only. This medication also has a toxic metabolite, norpropoxyphene, which can cause seizures (APS, 2009; Fine & Portnoy, 2007). Because of the potential for adverse effects, this medication is not recommended for use with older patients (APS; McLennon, 2005).

There are also some additional medications that should be avoided in the elderly. These medications fall into the category of mixed agonists-antagonist medications. They bind to the kappa site lower down on the spinal cord and have specific contraindications for the older patient. Indomethacin is an NSAID and amitriptyline is an antidepressant. All three medications listed below have undesirable side effects for the older patient.

- **Pentazocine (Talwin):** Delirium and agitation are two of the possible side effects of this mixed agonist-antagonist medication.

- **Indomethacin (Indocin):** This medication is for short-term use only, since it has the potential for central nervous system toxicity.

- **Amitriptyline (Elavil):** Anticholinergic effects and orthostatic hypotension are possible side effects of amitriptyline.

  (McLennon, 2005)

Coanalgesics

Coanalgesics, or adjuvant medications, enhance the analgesic effects of other pain medications but are more commonly used for other reasons. For example, antidepressants, most often used for treating depression (APS, 2009), may also be adjuvant medications for pain relief. The following different classes of medication can be used with good efficacy, especially for neuropathic pain:

- **Anticonvulsants**, such as carbamazepine, gabapentin, pregabalin, topiramate, and dilantin, are most commonly used for neuropathic pain or migraine headaches. Pregabalin has an FDA indication for diabetic neuropathy, fibromyalgia, and postherpetic neuralgia.

- **Antidepressants**, such as tricyclic antidepressants (TCAs), selective serotonin reuptake inhibitors (SSRIs), and serotonin norepinephrine reuptake inhibitors (SNRIs), also have a role in pain relief.

  - **TCAs:** Amitriptyline and other TCAs were used for neuropathic pain before the development of the gabalin medications. They are not recommended for use with older patients because of the potential for morning orthostatic hypotension, which increases the risk for falls.

  - **SSRIs:** SSRIs such as fluoxetine (Prozac) have mixed results with neuropathic pain relief.

  - **SNRIs:** Duloxetine (Cymbalta) is FDA-approved for use in treating diabetic neuropathy and fibromyalgia. The side effects of this

> **Clinical Tip**
>
> Because somnolence, dizziness, and sedation are common side effects for some of the coanalgesic medications, the dosing for older patients should be reduced when started and then slowly titrated upward.

medication are dose-related; starting with conservative doses and escalating carefully will make this medication tolerable for the older patient.

Venlafaxine (Effexor) is another SNRI that can be used as a coanalgesic. Since ECG changes were seen with venlafaxine, ECG monitoring is recommended for patients who are using this medication for adjuvant pain relief.

TARGETED TOPICAL ANALGESICS

A variety of topical agents can be used for adjuvant pain relief. Older patients tend to like these pain relief options because they are easy to use. The pain relief action is achieved through increased circulation to the painful area. Many of these medications are available over the counter, often at less cost than prescription medications, and come in a variety of strengths. Analgesic creams such as Ben Gay or Icy Hot have been very popular. In addition, the new topical patches with analgesic balms that can be applied to the painful area are easy to use. Other options include the following:

- **Lidocaine patches** (Lidoderm Patch 5%) are prescription-strength topical analgesic patches that were developed to treat postherpetic neuralgia (PHN). Athough only FDA-approved for PHN, the patches are used in the treatment of other conditions such as low back pain.

- **Capsaicin cream** (Zostrix) comes in two different strengths, 0.025% and 0.075%. Derived from hot peppers, capsaicin can be locally irritating, so wearing protective gloves when applying the cream is recommended. The cream needs to be applied regularly—up to four times daily for 2 weeks—before results can be seen. Capsaicin cream is used for neuropathic pain and is said to deplete Substance P, a neuropeptide produced at peripheral nerve endings that helps to facilitate pain signals to the central nervous system.

- **NSAID patches,** such as Flector, are topical patches designed to apply nonselective NSAIDs, such as diclofenac, directly over the area of pain. These may be used for mild to moderate pain of strains and sprains.

  (APS, 2009)

Breakthrough Pain

Pain is not static; rather, it is dynamic, with activity usually increasing its intensity (Dahl & Kehlet, 2006). For some patients, pain is present for the entire day but increases with activity such as preparing meals or making a trip to the health care provider. For these patients, an around-the-clock dosing or extended release medication may provide the least amount of variation in pain relief. However, with activity or at certain times of the day, patients may need extra medication, called *breakthrough medication,* to help control the pain. This should be a short-acting medication that accounts for a dose that is 5% to 15% of the total 24-hour dose, to be taken as needed as often as every 2 hours (APS, 2009).

For the older patient, activity is necessary to preserve functional status. It is important for older patients who are taking extended release medications to have supplemental doses of breakthrough medication available, so that they can participate in activity as needed. As with any opioid regimen for older patients, careful monitoring of side effects such as sedation is needed with patients who need extended release medication and use breakthrough doses for activity or sleep.

Issues with Medications Used for Pain

All opioids have the potential for side effects. Common side effects include constipation, sedation, or nausea and vomiting. Many of these side effects are time-limiting and will resolve over a period of 2 weeks or so, but others will not resolve, such as constipation. For the older patients, these side effects will limit the utility of pain medications and may cause the patient to discontinue taking the medication. In many of these cases, the patient prefers to stop taking the pain medication and suffer from pain, rather than tolerate the adverse effects of the medications.

- **Constipation:** A common side effect of opioid therapy, constipation is the only side effect that does not have tolerance. Patients who are on opioids should also be prescribed stool softeners and a laxative regimen. In addition, patients should be instructed to increase fluids and fiber in their diet. For patients who are not able to follow the required fluid intake recommendations, bulk laxatives are not indicated.

- **Sedation and respiratory depression:** Most commonly, sedation and respiratory depression occur at the beginning of opioid therapy. All patients should be observed for signs of sedation when they begin an opioid regimen. When other medications, that cause sedation, such as antiemetics, sleeping medications, or muscle relaxants, are used concomitantly, they should be used with caution and eliminated if they are not essential.

- **Pruritis:** Pruritis, or itching, may occur with opioids. It is the result of histamine release and is not a true allergy. To control the itching, an antihistamine such as diphenhydramine (Benadryl) or a medication such as hydroxizine (Atarax) can be used. These medications do, however, increase the potential for sedation when used concomitantly with opioids.

- **Nausea/vomiting:** Nausea and vomiting can be caused by pain medication or unrelieved pain. Antiemetics such as ondansetron (Zofran) or promethazine (Phenergan) can help to control the pain, but many are sedating.

  (D'Arcy, 2007)

Recommendations for using medication for pain control in older adults include

- Use shorter-acting medication at the onset of therapy to control adverse side effects.

- Reduce beginning opioid doses by 25% to 50% to decrease the potential for oversedation.

- For consistent pain, schedule medication to provide better pain relief and reduce the likelihood of needing increased doses for uncontrolled pain.

- Monitor older adults who are beginning opioid therapy at least daily, if not more frequently, since elimination of the drug may be affected by age-related liver and metabolic processing and other drugs the patient is taking.

- Avoid the following medications because of unwanted side effects and toxic metabolites: meperidine, propoxyphene, pentazocine, indomethacin, and amitriptyline.

  (McLennon, 2005)

Nursing Considerations for Older Patients

A baseline set of vital signs should be taken and documented for future reference. Using a baseline pain assessment and documenting any changes in pain intensity and functionality are critical for determining the success of the pain management interventions and medications, especially for older patients.

Make sure that the patient understands how to take opioid medications. Using a pillbox that can be filled by a friend or relative can help avoid unintentional duplicate medication administration. A frequent medication review is also indicated. Look at the medications the patient is taking and those that previously have been discontinued.

If the patient has independently stopped taking the medication, ask why and help to find a solution—whether it be a reduced dose, a laxative, or an alternate medication. All patients who are prescribed an opioid should start a laxative regimen consisting of a stool softener and mild laxative. Older patients fear constipation; by addressing the issue up-front, nonadherence related to constipation can be avoided.

Providing patients with education about their medications, including medication name, dose, time to take medication, and whom to call for questions, is an important aspect of pain management. This will avoid the "little blue pill" syndrome, wherein patients identify medication by pill size and color and do not know the name, dose, or use for the individual medications they take.

Summary

Using pain medication in older adults can be daunting, given the high likelihood of multidrug therapy and the high potential for adverse side effects. Opioids can effectively treat pain in the older adult, but using this type of medication means that more frequent monitoring and reassessment must be done. When treating pain in the older adult, remember that all patients have the right to have their pain assessed and treated adequately. Treating pain in older patients with opioids does require that more time be spent educating patients and monitoring medication usage and side effects, but it can be very rewarding to see these patients remain functional and have a good quality of life as they age.

Case Study

Sam Jones is a 79-year-old, retired train porter who is a patient in a primary care clinic where health care services are provided by the local university. In the clinic, he is seen by health care providers who are working on medical and advanced nursing degrees. There are many providers who rotate through the clinic in a year, so Sam does not have a consistent primary care physician or nurse practitioner. Sam keeps his appointment regularly. His main sources of income are Social Security and a railroad pension. He lives in an assisted living facility close to the clinic and has two children who accompany him to clinic visits.

Sam has a number of health care problems, including diabetes, hypertension, coronary artery disease, and peripheral vascular disease. In addition, he has minor vision and hearing impairments, for which he wears glasses and hearing aids. Recently, Sam has been complaining of a burning, painful numbness in his feet. He says the numbness is there all day, but gets much worse at night. He cannot sleep many nights, and the persistent pain is interfering with his daily walks. After a careful examination, his current health care provider diagnoses painful diabetic neuropathy (PDN). When Sam asks what can be done about the pain, the nurse practitioner says that a combination of medications can be useful. Sam receives prescriptions for a neuropathic pain medication and an opioid, but he can afford to fill only one of them, the gabapentin. He is ashamed to tell the provider that he cannot afford the medication that has been prescribed.

As Sam continues to complain about the foot pain, a new health care provider switches his medication to pregabalin, hoping for better effect, and raises the dose on the opioids. The pain is only slightly better at his next visit, so the provider again increases the opioid and prescribes an extended-release opioid medication for pain.

At Sam's next visit, the health care provider thinks that Sam may be asking for more opioids and may be misusing the drugs. She orders a urine screen, the results of which show that Sam has no opioids in his urine. When the provider asks Sam about the lack of opioid medication in his urine, he replies, "I really can't afford the drugs with all my other medications, and I don't really like taking them anyway. When I took them in the hospital the last time, they made me feel fuzzy-headed, and

I am afraid of becoming addicted to them. What should I do—not buy my heart and blood pressure medication and buy the pain medication instead? I need both, but I just can't afford it on my pension."

Critical Analysis Questions

1. Is Sam showing any signs of addiction? Opioid dependency? If not, why did the health care provider think he might be misusing his opioid medications?

2. Are the medication choices made for Sam's pain the best for his condition? If so, why?

3. What types of medications are most helpful when treating neuropathic pain?

4. Can older adults be treated with opioids, or do they need a milder type of pain medication?

5. Are NSAIDs a good medication choice for the older adult? If not, why?

4

COMPLEMENTARY METHODS FOR PAIN RELIEF

Older patients are often very comfortable with using complementary or nonpharmacologic methods for pain relief. They commonly try to treat minor pain complaints with home remedies—heat, cold, and medicinal rubs or creams that have proven helpful in the past. It is especially common for older patients with some form of musculoskeletal pain complaint, such as arthritis, to use a topical cream or heat to help relieve the pain (Khatta, 2007).

As with any type of treatment, it is best to use those that have the best research support with proven outcomes. Researchers at the National Institutes of Health (NIH) are studying alternative treatments and have formed a group called the National Center for Complementary and Alternative Medicine (NCCAM). This group of researchers is determining the validity of all types of complementary methods for adjunct pain relief, including supplements and herbal remedies, energy therapies, and treatments such as chiropractic manipulation and acupuncture.

The general term for these methods has been shortened to complementary and alternative medicine (CAM), which is defined as "a group of diverse medical and health care systems, practices, and products not presently considered to be a part of conventional medicine" (American Pain Society [APS], 2006). Put more simply, complementary pain relief techniques are meant to complement, not replace, mainstream medical therapeutics. If older patients are using complementary methods for pain relief, they often will not volunteer the information to their health care provider. Because some supplements and herbal remedies can interfere with mainstream medications, it is important to ask patients about any over-the-counter or other types of supplements they are taking. They may not even consider this information important, but for the health care provider, it can be an integral piece of the patient's history.

> ## Clinical Tip
>
> As part of any office visit, or history and physical, older patients should be questioned about nonpharmacologic interventions they are using for pain relief, including over-the-counter supplements and herbal remedies, therapies such as chiropractic, and home remedies.

CAM therapies are attractive options, because some older patients with chronic pain conditions do not like the side effects of pain medications. And, in some cases, they cannot afford the cost of pain medications. Older patients obtain information on these techniques and medications from a variety of sources. The January/February 2009 edition of *AARP the Magazine* includes a section on using CAM modalities to help relieve pain. Also, many older patients are very Internet-savvy—they go online and pick up bits of information that may be helpful or harmful, depending on the source (American Geriatrics Society [AGS], 2002). Older patients have many options when looking for information on a particular type of therapy.

Many Americans are open to using CAM therapies, and heating pads, cold wraps, analgesic balms, and other basic treatments for pain are commonly available in homes. In a 1993 survey, Americans reported that they made 629 million visits to CAM practitioners (Eisenberg, 1993). In Europe and Australia, estimates of the percentage of patients who use CAM therapies vary widely, ranging from about 20% to 70% (O'Hara, 2003). Many primary care practitioners do not ask patients if they use CAM therapies, but about 40% of patients volunteer this information (O'Hara). In a 2002 survey, NCCAM determined that the most common conditions for which patients used CAM were

- Back pain

- Neck pain

- Joint pain

- Arthritis

- Headache
  (Pierce, 2009)

TYPES OF CAM

Complementary and alternative medicine is a holistic, commonly used approach to pain relief for patients with chronic pain. Many of the therapies, such as acupuncture, are minimally invasive. Others, such as energy therapies of Reiki or Therapeutic Touch (TT), are noninvasive. Depending on how these therapies are used in the plan of care, there are three methods for incorporating CAM:

- **Complementary:** These techniques or therapies are used in conjunction with recognized mainstream medical practices—for example, acupuncture might be used concurrently with medication for low back pain.

- **Alternative:** With alternative medicine, the patient forgoes use of recognized medical therapy to treat a condition. For example, vitamin or herbal supplements might be used in place of radiation or chemotherapy for cancer treatment.

- **Integrative:** CAM practitioners have coined the term integrative medicine to describe the combined use of pharmacotherapy and nonpharmacologic methods for medical treatment. This term was popularized by Dr. Andrew Weil (O'Hara, 2003).
  (*National Center for Complementary and Alternative Medicine [NCCAM], 2004*)

A wide variety of complementary and alternative therapies is available. Some, such as heat or cold, are very simple to use, but others, such as biofeedback, require training. A trained practitioner might be necessary to administer other therapies, such as TT.

The NCCAM has defined four main types of CAM:

- **Body-based therapies,** such as heat, cold, massage, and acupuncture

- **Cognitive behavioral approaches or mind-body work,** such as relaxation, biofeedback, and imagery

- **Energy medicine,** including Reiki and Therapeutic Touch

- **Nutritional approaches** that incorporate use of herbs and vitamin supplements

BODY-BASED THERAPIES

Body-based therapies include massage, acupuncture, and heat/cold. These therapies focus on hands-on treatments. Some of these techniques can be performed by the patients, while others, such as acupuncture, require a trained professional.

Heat and Cold

Patients commonly use heat and cold before they seek treatment from health care providers for injuries such as strains and sprains. A Cochrane report found little support for using heat and cold applications to treat lower-back pain (D'Arcy, 2007; French, 2006). However, additional information demonstrates that using a heat wrap can increase *functionality.* (D'Arcy, 2007; French, 2006).

Clinical Tip

Founded in 1993, The Cochrane Collaboration was named after a British epidemiologist. The nonprofit organization aims to provide accurate, up-to-date information about the effects of health care to a global audience. Cochrane produces and disseminates systematic reviews of health care interventions and promotes the search for evidence in the form of clinical trials and other studies of interventions. The major product of the organization is the Cochrane Database of Systematic Reviews, published quarterly as part of *The Cochrane Library* (Cochrane Collaboration, n.d.).

Using a heating pad or hot pack can increase circulation to the affected area, decrease stiffness, reduce pain, and relieve muscle spasms (ASPMN, 2002). When using heat, be sure the patient has sensation to feel it and caution him or her to

- Use it for less than 30 minutes.

- Monitor use carefully over areas of decreased circulation to avoid burns.

- Avoid placing it over areas where mentholated creams have been used, which can increase the potential for skin damage.

- Never place heat over a patch delivering medications such as fentanyl, medications for hypertension, or smoking cessation patches. The heat over these patches will increase delivery of the medication to patients and put them at risk for overdose.

Ice baths, cold packs, or ice massages are helpful for decreasing the pain of sprains and strains, low back pain, and muscle spasms (ASPMN, 2002). Many older patients do not like the cold sensation and defer using the therapy, although it would be an effective adjunct for pain relief. The cold applications work by

- Decreasing nerve conduction

- Producing cutaneous counter-irritation

- Constricting blood flow

- Helping to relax muscles

- Reducing local and systemic metabolic activity
  (ASPMN, 2002)

RICE Therapy

RICE (rest, ice, compression, and elevation), a commonly used variation of cold therapy, has been used successfully for treating minor injuries (Berry, Covington, Dahl, Katz, & Miaskowski, 2006).

As with heat applications, cold packs should be used for short periods of time. Patients with de-sensitized skin, such as those with cardiovascular disease or diabetes, should carefully monitor the application sites for skin damage.

Acupuncture

One of the oldest CAM therapies, acupuncture, originated in China, where it was used to balance the yin and yang, or energy of life forces (O'Hara, 2003; ASPMN, 2002). The energy moves up and down in the body along meridians. When the energy flow is blocked, insufficient, or unbalanced, illness or pain can occur (Khatta, 2007). Using acupuncture can help restore balance to the body and open up the blocked energy.

There are several types of acupuncture, depending on the area of the world where it is being practiced. In most acupuncture practices, thin needles are inserted through the skin into acupuncture points (Dillard & Knapp, 2005; NCCAM, 2004). Once the needles are in place, they are manipulated by hand or electrically stimulated to release neurotransmitters that help to relieve pain (Dillard & Knapp).

Acupuncture has been used for centuries on many different types of patients, and with a wide variety of physical complaints. Patients with cancer, fibromyalgia, osteoarthritis, labor pain, and dental pain are all populations where acupuncture has been found to be beneficial (APS, 2005; Dillard & Knapp, 2005). A study of 570 patients with osteoarthritis who received acupuncture noted improvements in function and decreased pain levels (Khatta, 2007). In a review of therapy used for relief of lower-back pain, acupuncture and dry needling were found to be better than sham or no treatment for pain relief and improved function, but researchers recommended more focused studies on the technique (Furlan, Brosseau, Imamura, & Irvin, 2006.)

Massage

The NIH's National Center for Complementary and Alternative Medicine (2004) defines massage as pressing, rubbing, and otherwise manipulating muscles and soft tissues in the body. Some massage therapists use scented oils, such as lavender, or other compounds that are thought to further relax the body. The effect of massage is thought to be muscle relaxation and lengthening, which allow oxygen and increased blood flow into the affected area. Older patients may enjoy this form of therapy and can benefit if cost is not prohibitive (Bruckenthal & D'Arcy, 2007).

Other Types of Body-Based Therapies

Not all forms of body-based therapies are well supported by research. The findings for chiropractic, for example, are not well established. However, there is some good evidence that chiropractic therapy is effective for chronic or subacute low back pain (Chou & Huffman, 2007).

Therapies with little solid research support include the use of magnets and copper bracelets.

However, those therapies that do have support can be useful to help relieve pain. For example, physical therapy for reconditioning and improving balance can help to maintain the mobility and functionality of older patients (AGS, 2002; Bruckenthal & D'Arcy, 2007). A regular physical therapy program has been found to reduce pain and improve mood (Bruckenthal & D'Arcy). If the program is individualized to the patient's ability, the patient should be able to perform at a level where improvements are possible.

Cognitive Behavioral Therapy

For patients with intact cognitive functions, complementary methods such as relaxation, biofeedback, self-hypnosis, and imagery can provide additional pain relief (AGS, 2002; D'Arcy). Not all older patients are open to trying these techniques, but for patients who are, these techniques can be a useful adjunct and provide a needed element in controlling the condition.

Relaxation

Several different types of relaxation techniques can help control pain (Cole & Brunk, 1999). The various levels and types of relaxation techniques include the following:

- Regulation of breathing which can lead to decreased respiratory efforts

- Relaxation tapes

- Relaxation exercises
  (D'Arcy, 2007)

These techniques reduce physical tension and promote muscle relaxation and emotional well-being (NCCAM, 2004). Relaxation is beneficial for patients who have chronic pain or cancer pain, as well as for surgical patients (Dillard & Knapp, 2005). Major benefits of relaxation techniques include an improved sense of well-being and higher scores on quality of life scales (Dillard & Knapp).

Imagery

Imagery is a form of relaxation in which patients are encouraged to form a mental image of a peaceful, soothing place (D'Arcy, 2007). They are asked to "feel" the place, smell it, taste it, and enjoy the feeling of comfort that the scenario provides (ASPMN, 2002). Patients can create the mental pictures themselves, or recorded images can be used if patients have difficulty developing the mental images. Some older patients are not receptive to this technique; they find it difficult to relax, provide an image, and work with it to create the scenario.

For example, a patient could be asked to relax and picture a beautiful red rose. The exercise continues as the patient is asked to smell the rose; see the exquisite, rich color; and feel the soft petals of the flower. This image is peaceful and pleasant. By using such an image, a patient can learn to relax and picture the image when they feel pain or stress.

The Arthritis Self Management Program (ASMP) uses some mind-body techniques (AGS, 2002). These include

- Education

- Cognitive restructuring

- Physical activity

- Problem solving

- Relaxation

- Development of communication skills to help interact with health care professionals

This program demonstrated reduced pain that lasted over a 4-year time period and resulted in a cost savings of four to five times the cost of the program (Khatta, 2007).

Biofeedback, hypnosis, and meditation are other forms of relaxation techniques. Studies have found that meditation can reduce pain and help patients with chronic pain learn to cope more effectively (Khatta, 2007). All the techniques have research support for their use; which technique works for a specific patient depends on the type of approach the patient prefers (O'Hara, 2003).

ENERGY THERAPIES

Energy healing is derived from the concept of qigong, an external and internal energy control technique that has been a part of Asian cultures for many centuries. Newer energy therapies include Reiki, TT, and Healing Touch (Pierce, 2009). Although there are differences in practices, the therapies have the following similarities:

- The human body has an energy field that is generated from within the body to the outer world.

- A universal energy flows through all living things.

- Self-healing is promoted through the free-flowing energy field.

- Disease and illness may be felt in the energy field and can be changed by the healing intent of the practitioner.
  (Pierce, 2009)

Energy therapies can help relax the patient and provide pain relief. Two of the most commonly practiced therapies are TT and Reiki.

Reiki

In 1914, Japanese Buddhist monk Mikao Usui began developing and teaching the techniques used by Reiki practitioners (Pierce, 2009). Practitioners use the natural energy of the universe to release blockage in points within a patient's body. The configuration of hand placement for Reiki uses chakras, or energy points. Reiki practitioners channel the energy of the universe through their hands into the chakras, easing blocked points. In this technique, Reiki practitioners transmit energy either over long distances or by directly placing hands on the patients (NCCAM, 2005).

There are three levels of Reiki practice. In the basic level, energy blockages are identified and opened. This process allows patients to feel relaxed and experience emotional and physical healing. The Reiki practitioner who channels energy for the patient also receives benefit and may feel more relaxed and in tune with his or her own body energy after the session is completed. In Reiki, the second level and master level add more complex energy channeling and include the process of transferring energy over long distance.

Studies to determine the benefit of Reiki have focused on patients with cancer. In a study of 24 cancer patients using Reiki or rest periods, the Reiki patients had a significant decrease in pain (Pierce, 2009).

Therapeutic Touch

Therapeutic Touch originated in the 1970s as a collaboration between Dolores Krieger and Dora Kunz, who hoped that the practice of energy healing could become part of standard nursing procedures (Pierce, 2009). Unfortunately, the practice remains a nonstandard addition to patient care, although it is popular in some areas of the country.

Therapeutic Touch is a form of energy medicine in which the practitioner does not touch the patient receiving the therapy, but rather focuses the energy on the patient's aura. Often it is mistakenly referred to as "laying on of hands." The premise of TT is that the practitioner's healing force transfers or channels energy, thereby positively affecting the recovery of the patient (NCCAM, 2005). As the TT practitioner allows his or her hands to move over the patient, blocked energy is identified, and healing forces are directed to the area to promote healing and pain relief.

Some studies indicate greater pain relief with the use of TT in patients with chronic pain and fibromyalgia, when compared to patient groups not receiving the energy treatment option (Pierce, 2009). However, because randomized, placebo-controlled studies are difficult with TT, it is hard to measure the true effect of the practice.

Energy therapies are controversial, because there is little conventional research support. Members of the NCCAM group are undertaking research into the use of Reiki and TT, and some of the early work is showing promise.

Nutritional Approaches

Folk literature is full of remedies to heal and cure, and herbal remedies are among the most common forms of complementary therapeutics (Khatta, 2007). They are simple and easy to use; are viewed as noninvasive and benign (not always true), with few side effects; and unfortunately, have little or no quality control mechanism. Between 1990 and 1997, herbal remedy use increased by 380%, and the annual expenditure on herbal remedies in the United States exceeded 1.5 billion dollars (Khatta).

In the early years of the United States, barkers and peddlers sold folk remedies from town to town. Naturally, there was no quality control on these products, and the buyers were never sure what they were purchasing. Now, dietary supplements are categorized under the Dietary Supplement Health and Education Act (DSHEA) of 1994, which requires quality, safety, and efficacy standards. Even today, buyers should be wary and consult with their primary care provider before using supplements and herbs. This is especially true for pregnant and compromised patients such as those with immunosuppression.

Some common herbal remedies include the following:

- **Cayenne (Capsicum):** Cayenne can be made in plasters and placed over the painful areas. Capsaicin, the active ingredient of cayenne (Khatta, 2007), is sold as an over-the-counter cream. It has a burning, stinging sensation when applied as a cream. The use of capsaicin requires three to four applications daily over at least 2 weeks to see any improvement. When applying capsaicin cream, patients should wear gloves and avoid touching other parts of the body, especially the eyes.

- **Devil's claw (Harpagophytum procumbens):** Use of this herb in patients with osteoarthritis may result in a reduction in pain levels and an increase in mobility (Khatta, 2007).

- **Willow bark (Salix alba):** Results for use of this herb are inconsistent, and only short-term improvement has been demonstrated (Khatta, 2007).

- **Corydalis:** A frequently used herb, Corydalis is an alkaloid with potent analgesic properties (Dillard & Knapp, 2005). Traditionally, it has been used for menstrual pain.

Nutritional supplements include the following:

- **Glucosamine and chondroitin:** Studies have shown that the use of glucosamine and chondroitin results in a delay of disease progression over time, and that combination medications can reduce pain in osteoarthritis patients (Khatta, 2007).

- **Omega-3 fatty acids:** Omega-3 fatty acids affect prostaglandin metabolism, which is associated with the inflammatory process. Studies have shown that fish oil has anti-inflammatory effects in patients with rheumatoid arthritis, whereas flaxseed oil has not had similar effects (Khatta, 2007).

Clinical Tip

Because nutritional supplements can interact with mainstream medications, health care providers should ask all patients if they are taking a supplement or herbal remedy. Only supplements and herbs that have shown efficacy in clinical trials and are recommended by the NCCAM should be used for complementary pain relief.

Summary

There are many types of nonpharmacologic therapies that patients find helpful, including music, storytelling, humor, and distraction. Most of these therapies are benign and offer positive support for the medical regimen. Since there are many of these therapies to choose from, patients can usually find a treatment to complement their conventional therapy.

Case Study

Mrs. Stone, 76, is an older neighbor of yours. She usually is very active with gardening, going to meetings at the senior center, and visiting her grandchildren. Mrs. Stone's daughter tells you her mother has not been feeling well. Because Mrs. Stone has a cardiac condition, you ask if she is having difficulty with her heart. Her daughter replies that her mother's cardiac condition is very stable; the problem is more to do with her osteoarthritis, which has caused chronic pain in her shoulders, hips, and knees. Despite large amounts of acetaminophen and mentholated creams, Mrs. Stone cannot get a good night's sleep, and she either wanders the house at night or sleeps in a reclining chair. She is very depressed about her condition and misses her friends and family. Her daughter says, "If mom doesn't start feeling better soon, she may have to sell her house and move in with me. I know it would devastate her, but she really needs some help." You ask what Mrs. Stone has been using for pain relief, and her daughter replies, "Some sort of herbal supplement for the depressed mood, another for sleep, and a lot of over-the-counter acetaminophen and ibuprofen. Mom doesn't like to take strong medication, because it makes her fuzzy-headed."

Critical Analysis Questions

1. Are herbal supplements the best choice for Mrs. Stone to use for depression and sleep?

2. Are there complementary methods that might help Mrs. Stone decrease her pain and impaired functionality?

3. Are the over-the-counter medications she's taking the best choice for Mrs. Stone, given her cardiac condition and possible side effects from the medications?

4. What are the overall effects of chronic pain on Mrs. Stone?

5. Do you think Mrs. Stone would be better off if she just gave in and moved in with her daughter?

5

Acute Pain Management

Acute pain is very different from chronic pain or neuro-pathic pain. The purpose of acute pain is to warn the body that it has been injured, and the pain gradually diminishes as the injury resolves (American Pain Society, 2009; American Society for Pain Management Nursing, 2006).

Most acute pain is the result of surgery or injuries such as falls, sprains, and muscle strains. Patients who have surgery expect to have some pain for a short time after the surgery. The problem for older patients is that they may lack the physical reserves needed to recover from an acute injury. The debilitating effects of acute pain can lead to a change in lifestyle, loss of quality of life, and the end of an enjoyable life as they know it.

Older patients who have acute pain vary widely in their abilities and health status. Some individuals are healthy and unimpaired, even at very old ages. These people likely exercise regularly, control their diet, and enjoy hobbies. Others who are experiencing acute pain have multiple comorbidities and medications. These patients often cannot exercise regularly and have limitations on their functionality. They also may be obese. Still other older patients may have dementia or episodes of delirium while hospitalized.

Nurses who care for older patients in an acute care setting should be aware of some of the variation in patient types and differences in treatment and patient care required. Taking care of patients who have dementia and are unable to report pain can be challenging. And, community-dwelling patients in long-term settings can be at risk for acquiring drug-resistant bacterial infections and may be less active, which results in deconditioning and impaired skin integrity. Nutritional deficits for many older patients can impact the healing and recovery process, creating the need for an extended stay in a hospital or skilled-care facility.

ACUTE PAIN IN OLDER PATIENTS

Older patients who fall or undergo surgery have completely different needs from their younger counterparts. Younger patients have better physical reserves and shorter recovery times. Older patients who are deconditioned, or who have visual or hearing impairments, may require more assistance and reconditioning through physical therapy to resume their daily activities.

Treatment of any kind of acute pain in older patients begins with a thorough assessment, either in the emergency department (ED) or in the surgical pre-testing/pre-holding area. The health care provider must determine the severity of the pain, its duration, and its cause. Has the pain worsened, interrupted sleep, or spread to a new area? What is the patient using to self-treat the pain? Be sure to have the patient or a family member provide a list of all medications the patient is currently taking, including over-the-counter medications, herbal supplements, and vitamins. Confirm the medication, dose, and length of time the patient has been on the medication with the patient, family member, or nursing facility. Also, find out who is prescribing the medication. Make sure that all medications that are no longer being taken are eliminated from current medication lists. Also, if possible, determine how often pain medications that were ordered to be taken "as needed" are being used. This is particularly important for opioid medications; if they have been ordered but have not been given regularly, the patient should be considered opioid-naïve.

In 2001, the Joint Commission on Accreditation of Healthcare Organizations (JCAHO), now the Joint Commission, issued the following standards for pain management:

- Patients have the right to have their pain assessed and reassessed regularly.

- Patients have the right to have their pain treated adequately.

- There should be no barriers to pain assessment, such as a patient's foreign language or nonverbal status.

- Pain should not interfere with rehabilitation.

- Patients should be involved in planning their care.

- Patients should have access to pain specialists, if needed (JACHO, 2000).

A newer recommendation from the Joint Commission indicates that each patient should be assessed according to his or her specific condition and ability. This will affect the assessment process for older adults, as some older patients have aphasia, dementia, or other conditions that make assessment and treatment of pain more difficult. The most current recommendations can be found on the Joint Commission website at www.jointcommision.org.

Older Patients in the Emergency Department

Older patients most commonly visit the emergency department (ED) for treatment resulting from an injury or accident. In a review of ED admissions, pain was the main complaint for 52.2% of patients (Cordell et al., 2002). For older patients, pain may be the reason for an ED visit, but a comorbidity such as arthritis, low back pain, or a neuropathic pain condition may also be present. In addition, painful procedures may be performed as diagnostic tests or treatment options, including

- Nasogastric intubation

- Incision and drainage of abscesses

- Fracture reduction

- Urethral catheterization

  (Singer, Richman, Kowalska, & Thode, 1999)

A review by Singer and colleagues (1999) of ED records found that local anesthetics were used before these painful procedures only 12.8% of the time. The use of pain medication in EDs is also relatively low (56%), the wait for medication can be very long (more than 2 hours), and pain medication doses can be suboptimal (32%; Singer et al.). When older patients who are in pain come into the ED, the chances of getting adequate and effective pain relief are not promising. For non-verbal patients, the chances of getting pain medication would be even less likely.

To make a visit to the ED easier and more beneficial, older patients should have the following items ready:

- A list of all current medications, with medication dose and time last taken. The long-term facility or acute care facility where the patient has been living may provide this list.

- A list of allergies to medications, along with the type of reaction the patient had to the medication.

- The phone number of the patient's primary health care provider, where records are located.

- The phone number of a family member and the person or persons who hold power of attorney for health care decisions.

- A copy of advance directives that lists the power of attorney for health care decisions and that documents treatment preferences.

Falls account for a high number of ED visits by older patients. In 2003, more than 1.8 million adults age 65 or older were treated in EDs for falls, and 421,000 were hospitalized (Clayton, 2008). The fall rate is highest among patients in the over-85 age group (Clayton). The ability to function, live independently, and have a worthwhile quality of life can deteriorate very quickly after a fall. One important consideration is that 50% of older adults who fall and who were ambulating before the fall do not recover their previous level of mobility (Clayton). Falls also account for 40% of nursing home admissions (Clayton).

To determine whether older patients are at risk of falling, consider the following indicators of increased risk:

- Being more than 65 years old (higher if more than 75 years old)

- Being female (the rate of falls in women is two to three times that of men)

- Being housebound

- Having the genetic predisposition for poor bone structure

- Living alone

- Smoking

- Drinking to excess

  (Clayton, 2008)

As people age, the natural result is a loss of hearing, vision, and other natural means of preserving safety when walking. Moreover, balance can be affected by medications and chronic conditions such as Parkinson's disease. The following basic safety tenets help ensure a safe environment for older adults and decrease the likelihood of falls:

- Remove any loose area rugs or extension cords.

- Make sure the patient knows how to use mobility aids such as canes and walkers.

- Keep the patient's clothing simple and well-fitting; no loose, flowing robes.

- Make sure the patient wears glasses and a hearing aid, if needed.

  (Clayton, 2008)

Older Patients in the Surgical Area

Approximately 90% of hip fractures are related to falls (Clayton, 2008). In 2000, 350,000 patients, mainly women, were treated for fall-related hip fractures (Clayton). By 2050, the number of hip fractures is expected to reach 650,000 annually. The personal loss and wide-reaching effects of these falls that result in hip fractures cannot truly be measured. When a person falls, additional injuries such as closed head injuries, other fractures, or soft tissue injuries may be present. These ancillary injuries can slow rehabilitation and create a need for more medical interventions, such as surgery.

When an older patient is confined to bed for an extended period of time during recovery, muscle disuse can lead to deconditioning that requires a complete physical therapy regimen to reverse. Patients can lose the ability to function independently and may need to take medications with side effects that can cause further delays in recovery. Lung function is compromised with extended bed rest, and the potential for pneumonia increases. These conditions increase the probability of extended recovery time and additional interventions, such as antibiotics or longer rehabilitation times.

The indicated treatment for hip fracture is either joint replacement or hip pinning, if replacement is not possible. When older patients are having a procedure such as a joint replacement, abdominal surgery, or other types of elective surgery, the nurse caring for them should realize that older patients are at higher risk for complications during and after surgery (Clayton, 2008). The following risk factors and long-term lifestyle choices can affect how well the older patient tolerates surgery and what outcomes are achieved:

- Smoking

- Alcohol abuse

- Obesity

- Deconditioning due to sedentary lifestyle

- Dietary deficiencies, such as low fruit and vegetable intake
  (Clayton)

When the older patient is scheduled for surgery, a complete preoperative evaluation is needed to assess any factors that could lead to an increased risk for mortality. These factors include

- Nutritional status, especially hydration status

- Recent weight changes

- Chronic health problems such as arthritis, urinary tract infections, hypertension, and hearing and vision loss

- Medications of all types

- Skin integrity
  (Clayton, 2008)

When older patients have surgery, reducing their anxiety and fear plays a large role in making the experience successful. Educating patients about what is happening and what they can expect helps to reassure them about the surgery. Family members also can reassure the patient about the surgical experience. Pain is part of the injury and recovery process. A comprehensive plan of care will help provide older patients with the best potential for returning to their pre-hospital functionality.

POSTOPERATIVE PAIN MANAGEMENT

Why do older patients have such poor pain management in the acute postoperative setting? Common reasons for poor pain management in this age group include

- Failure of health care providers to assess pain

- Inadequate knowledge about pain assessment and management

- Misperception that pain is a natural and expected consequence of aging

- Belief that pain should be expected after surgery

- Concern about using analgesics with patients who have cognitive dysfunction or other comorbid illnesses
  (Karani & Meier, 2004)

After surgery, patients need to have their pain assessed, reassessed, and adequately treated. The American Society of PeriAnesthesia Nurses (ASPAN) has a pain and comfort guideline that many post-anesthesia units use to implement best practices in pain relief in the immediate postoperative time period (ASPAN, 2003). The guideline focuses on using pain medications and complementary methods for pain relief. Complementary methods that are recommended include the use of heat, cold, and music (ASPAN).

Opioids are most often used in the postoperative period for patients with injuries and surgical procedures that cause severe pain. If the pain experienced by an older patient is not too severe, opioids might not be the best fit for pain control. Older patients can certainly use opioids, but the medication will need dose adjustments and careful monitoring for side effects.

Opioid doses for older patients should be reduced by 25% to 50%, depending on the overall condition of the patients. Opioid medications have a higher profile for side effects such as hallucinations, delirium, or constipation. Changing the opioid may resolve these effects, and the new opioid can be continued.

Short-acting pain medications and combination medications such as oxycodone APAP or hydrocodone APAP may be used intermittently or scheduled around-the-clock, if needed. Be aware of possible liver toxicity because these drugs contain acetaminophen. Older patients who are opioid-naïve should be observed carefully for sedation, nausea, and feelings of dizziness/mental clouding. Any patient who receives an opioid for pain control should be on a laxative regimen, since all opioids are constipating. If patients are nauseated, the nurse should be aware that the sedating effects of opioids are increased when an anti-emetic with sedating effect is added. Although opioids often are blamed for over-sedation, the cause may be the result of a combination of medications: opioid, anti-emetic, sleeping medication, or antihistamine for pruritis.

The intramuscular (IM) route of medication administration is no longer recommended for pain medication, because the rate of absorption cannot be controlled and tissue can scleros (APS, 2009).

Especially with an older patient who has less muscle mass, less adipose tissue, and thinner dermis, the intravenous route of medication administration is preferred if the oral route is not possible.

A patient-controlled analgesia (PCA) machine is a good option for pain control in the postoperative period, if patients understand how to use it. Older patients who are cognitively impaired are not good candidates for this patient-activated pain management technique.

The PCA medication delivery system consists of a small pump that provides opioid pain medication according to a preset prescription to the patient's IV access. When patients experience pain, they can push the button and receive a dose of medication. This allows patients to stay ahead of the pain. Many patients like using this system for pain relief after surgery or injury, because it allows them to deliver a dose of pain medication without having to wait for the nurse to bring the medication and administer it.

The key to success with PCA is correct patient selection. The Joint Commission and the Institute for Safe Medication Practices (ISMP) have identified the types of patients who are not good candidates for PCA:

- Infants and young children

- Confused older adults

- Patients who are obese, have sleep apnea, or have asthma or other respiratory-related comorbidities that could contribute to the potential for over-sedation.

- Patients taking sedating medication such as muscle relaxants, antiemetics, and sleeping medication, as they can potentiate the sedating effects of opioids.

  (Cohen, 2006; Cohen & Smetzer, 2005; D'Arcy, 2007)

Two additional issues need to be considered when determining if an older patient is a good candidate for PCA. First, basal rates are no longer considered safe for opioid-naïve patients—the rationale being that the additional medication does not enhance pain relief, but creates a higher potential for over-sedation (APS, 2009). The second safety issue to consider is PCA by proxy—that is, someone other than the patient pushing the PCA button. Once pain is controlled, the patient may fall sleep and not push the button. If another person pushes the button, he or she may inadvertently overdose the patient. For this reason, a patient who cannot activate the PCA is not a good candidate for this option for medication delivery. One case of death through PCA by proxy has been documented; recommendations from the Joint Commission and ISMP do not endorse PCA by proxy. If ever used, there should be strict orders, criteria, and regulations on the activation of the button.

In many situations, such as flail chest, multiple broken ribs, and thoracotomy surgery, an epidural catheter with local anesthetic or an opioid such as fentanyl may provide excellent pain relief. With epidural analgesia, a needle is inserted so a catheter can be inserted into the epidural space at the level of the injury or surgery (see Figure 5.1).

The nurse programs a small infusion pump, following the prescriber's orders for dose, dose interval, and the total amount the patient can use in a 1-hour time period. This technique, recommended by the American Society of Anesthesiologists (ASA; Ashburn, Caplan, Carr, Connis, Ginsberg et al., 2004), can provide a high level of pain relief with a small amount of opioids. Patients as old as 100, or older, can tolerate an epidural and benefit from the pain relief. Physical limitations to using an epidural catheter in older patients include a spinal malformation, anticoagulant therapy, or previous surgeries to the area where the catheter would need to be placed.

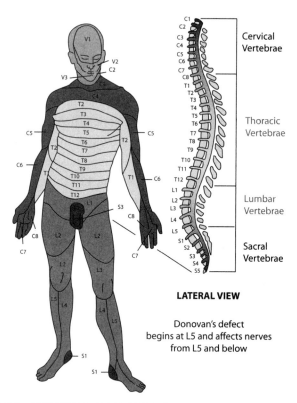

FIGURE 5.1   EPIDURAL ANALGESIA CAN BE GIVEN AT THE CREVICAL,
THORACIC, LUMBAR, OR SACRAL AREAS, DEPENDING ON THE
LEVEL OF INJURY

If opioids cannot be used for an older patient, what other pain relief
options are available? ASA (Ashburn et al., 2004) suggests intraoperative
blocks for adjunct pain relief. Performed during surgery, intraoperative blocks can provide pain relief for a period of 6 to 8 hours after the
procedure. Using a local anesthetic such as bupivacaine, a block can
be placed along a nerve, such as a femoral nerve block, or in specific
areas, such as intercostal blocks in the rib area (Ashburn et al.). A local
anesthetic pump (see Figure 5.2) can provide continuous analgesia for
several days, if it is combined with an external reservoir that delivers the
local anesthetic at a preset rate.

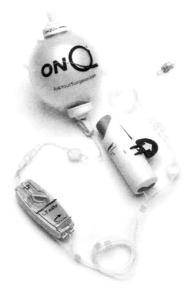

FIGURE 5.2   EXAMPLE OF A LOCAL ANESTHETIC PUMP

Patients with total joint replacements who use the combination of continuous local anesthetic nerve block with a PCA report greater satisfaction and have decreased length of stay, greater mobility, and fewer opioid-related side effects (Idelli, Grant, Neilsen, Parker, 2005).

An intraoperative block can be particularly helpful for older patients, since this approach offers an alternative to opioids. A combination of intraoperative block and low-dose opioids can help older patients recover more quickly and improve their ability to participate in physical therapy, which results in improved functionality.

DELIRIUM/DEMENTIA

Delirium can occur when older patients are hospitalized, receive a variety of medications for surgery, and use opioids for pain relief in the postoperative period. Delirium is a sudden-onset, confusional state that occurs in approximately 10% to 60% of hospitalized patients, with older patients developing the condition more frequently than younger patients (Vaurio, Sands, Wang, Mullen, Leung, 2006).

The risk factors for delirium include the following:

- Older age, patients older than 65 years of age

- Environmental factors (e.g., ICU admission, surgery)

- Inadequate pain relief

- Medical conditions (e.g., infections, decreased renal or hepatic clearance)

- Medications—polypharmacy or suddenly stopping a medication

- Impaired nutritional/fluid status, such as dehydration and malnutrition

  (Gray-Vickrey, 2005)

Delirium/Dementia

Delirium

Delirium is defined as an acute disorder of attention and cognition (Gray-Vickrey, 2005; Inouye, Van Dyk, Alessi, Balkin, Siegal et al., 1990).

Dementia

Dementia is a cognitive impairment that is a chronic, progressive condition with slow onset and indefinite duration (ASPMN, 2006).

In a study of 333 postoperative patients older than 74 years of age, 46% developed delirium (Vaurio et al., 2006). In an attempt to determine the cause of the delirium, pain scores, contributing factors, and pain medications were studied. Oral combination opioid medications were used in 64.6% of patients (the majority of those patients received a type of pure opioid mu agonist medication), and 32.2% of the patients received antihistamines.

Other medication-related predictors of delirium include the following:

- Preoperative pain at rest

- Preoperative pain with movement

- Pain at rest on postoperative day 1

- Use of oral opioids on postoperative day 1

- Use of benzodiazepines postoperatively

- Use of miscellaneous central nervous system medications
  (Vaurio et al., 2006)

When considering the most significant factors in the development of postoperative delirium, the study revealed that patients who experience severe preoperative pain, use an IV PCA, and receive neuraxial analgesia (an epidural) were equally at risk to develop postoperative delirium. Patients who used oral opioids, however, tended to have less risk for delirium.

In contrast to delirium, dementia is a cognitive impairment that slowly develops over time. Patients with dementia may not be able to express the pain they are feeling. Horgas, McLennon, and Floetke (2003) report that pain tolerance is significantly increased in patients with dementia, when compared to unimpaired older adults. Huffman and Kunik (2000) state that older adults with dementia may perceive pain differently. These findings indicate that, in cognitively impaired older adults,

- There may be higher pain thresholds and diminished warning.

- There is no difference between peripheral pain sensation or transmission of pain.

- Central nervous system changes may affect how the pain is interpreted.

For More Information

Chapter 2 discusses assessing cognitively impaired patients with behavioral pain scales; Chapter 3 describes pain medications that can be used with older patients; and Chapter 6 describes treating pain in patients with dementia.

Thus, despite the presence of pain, older patients with dementia may be unable to report what they are experiencing (Horgas et al., 2003). Pain that is not reported may not be treated. Studies show that patients with dementia receive significantly less medication than nonimpaired older patients with similar painful conditions (Horgas et al.).

An assessment using behavioral indicators and trials of pain medication may help health care providers to discover what relieves the pain in these individuals, which will help to ensure that delirious and demented patients receive adequate pain relief when hospitalized. Treating pain effectively in a cognitively impaired patient requires a good assessment of the patient, followed by a medication trial or appropriate intervention and a reassessment (Horgas et al., 2003).

SUMMARY

Most patients who are older than 65 have experienced some type of acute pain, whether from injury or surgery. Many health care providers are reluctant to uses opioid medication to treat acute pain for these patients, but since pain may be severe, it is important to develop a comfort level when treating these patients who have an acute onset of pain. It is also wise to remember that older patients may be cognitively impaired or delirious, but they still require adequate pain relief. Providing the older adult patient who has acute pain with adequate pain relief can result in a faster recovery, decreased length of stay after surgery, and increased functionality.

CASE STUDY

Frieda Jones is an 85-year-old woman living in an assisted living facility. She has mild memory problems, osteoarthritis, osteoporosis, and mild hypertension, but she can care for herself and enjoys the company of the other residents at the facility. She participates in activities such as card games on a daily basis, and she enjoys going on field trips provided by the assisted care facility. Frieda has three children who live locally and visit her often.

One night, Frieda got up to use the bathroom and fell. She couldn't get up right away, but was able to activate her emergency bathroom button. Staff who responded to the call found Frieda in severe pain, with her right leg externally rotated. She was transferred to the hospital by ambulance and told she had a fractured hip.

That night, Frieda was admitted to the orthopedic unit, where she was given morphine intravenously for her pain, which she rated as 7 on a 10-point scale. When the morning nurse arrived to do her pre-operative assessment, Frieda reported seeing water running down the walls and complained about being awakened so early in the morning. She wanted to know when they would leave for the field trip to the arboretum. When asked about her pain, Frieda could not provide a number. She told the nurse that she hurt, but she could not localize the pain to her hip.

Critical Analysis Questions

1. Is Frieda delirious or demented?
2. What type of pain control would be better for Frieda, e.g., have fewer side effects?
3. In the postoperative recovery period, would a PCA be a good option for Frieda?
4. Should Frieda be identified as a patient who is at risk for a fall? If so, what criteria apply? Does she need restraints?
5. Should Frieda be able to describe her pain and localize it? How will you know that Frieda has pain, if she can't tell you about it? Should she be medicated for pain if her assessment indicated a pain level requiring intervention?

6

CHRONIC PAIN
MANAGEMENT

Chronic pain is one of the most invasive and destructive pain conditions among the elderly. It can rob older patients of quality of life and the ability to function independently. The American Geriatrics Society (2002) reports that 25% to 50% of community-dwelling elders experience chronic pain; an estimated 45% to 80% of elders in long-term care experience chronic, daily pain.

Because chronic pain is so common among older patients, the health care system should be designed to assist and treat these patients. However, the real picture is that chronic pain among older patients is often ignored, underappreciated, or undertreated by health care providers (D'Arcy, 2008b). Although chronic pain is not limited to older patients, they may suffer more from debilitating chronic illnesses and injuries, compared to their younger counterparts because of comorbidities, depleted physical resilience, and diminished physical capacity.

By the year 2030, 20% of the population will be over the age of 65, according to predictions (Smeltzer, Bare, Hinkle, & Cheever, 2007). An increasing number of older patients with chronic pain will need attention from the health care system.

Older patients are subject to a number of chronic pain conditions that continue to progress as they age. Common chronic pain conditions include

- Vertebral compression fractures from osteoporosis

- Skin breakdown as a result of reduced mobility

- Poor circulation from impaired mobility or various chronic disease processes, such as atherosclerosis

- Osteoarthritis

- Postherpetic neuralgia

- Post-stroke pain

- Diabetic neuropathy

- Fractures

- Injury from falls

- Trigeminal neuralgia

- Headaches

  (Adapted from ASPMN, 2002)

As patients age and the number of patients in need of care for chronic pain conditions increases, the demand for care may very well outstrip the available resources. Additionally, older patients can suffer from a number of chronic pain conditions, not just a single complaint, which can lead to increased pain and decreased quality of life.

UNDERTREATMENT OF CHRONIC PAIN

Undertreatment of chronic pain in older adults is common. Health care providers fear using medications, such as opioids, that they perceive as having more risks than benefits for the older patient. Fear of addiction is a common finding among both patients and health care providers. In a survey on medication use in older patients, one in five older patients reported taking pain medications only occasionally during a 1-week period of time (Reyes-Gibby, Aday, Todd, Cleeland, & Anderson, 2007). This lack of seeking pain relief may result from health care providers who underprescribe medication, financial constraints, or the reluctance of older patients to take pain medications. The continued undertreatment of pain can cause

- Depression

- Anxiety

- Decreased socialization

- Sleep disturbances

- Impaired ambulation

- Increased health care utilization and costs

  (Bruckenthal & D'Arcy, 2007)

For More Information

The coupling of depression, emotional pain, and physical pain leads to statistically increased rates of suicide in older patients (Valente, 2008). Older patients with chronic pain should be screened for hopeless and helpless feelings, social isolation, and worsening depression, which can lead to suicide (Valente).

One result of the undertreatment of chronic pain in older adults, which previously was rarely addressed, is suicide (Valente, 2008). When patients feel like the pain will not end and medications do not decrease the pain, they can become depressed. Financial constraints can also make it difficult for older patients to obtain the pain medication they need. The pain from physical causes can be exacerbated by the emotional suffering that chronic pain can produce. The loss of function, independent living and ability to perform self-care can produce feelings of loss and grief.

In today's diverse society, older members of minority groups face increased risks for undertreated pain. A study of pain among minority patients indicated that 28% of community-dwelling minority patients reported daily pain (Reyes-Gibby, Aday, Todd, Cleeland, & Anderson, 2007; D'Arcy, 2008a). In an ethnically diverse population, predictors of severe pain include the following:

- Being a Medicaid recipient

- Having two or more comorbidities

- Having a low educational level

- Having psychological distress
  (D'Arcy, 2008a; Reyes-Gibby et al., 2007)

Regardless of the source of the pain condition, financial resources, or ability of the older adult to communicate, pain should be addressed in all health evaluations. Older patients should be encouraged to report unrelieved pain. If older patients have pain, clinicians should prescribe adequate pain relief medications and options. It is incumbent on all health care providers to make serious efforts to control chronic pain in older patients.

As mentioned in Chapter 1, myths can help foster undertreatment of pain in older patients. One myth is that pain is just a normal part of aging—older patients should just "get used" to having daily pain. With the proper knowledge base and judicious use of medications, pain can be effectively treated in older patients. Using doses that will not increase sedation or cause side effects such as nausea, dizziness, or constipation can help the patient effectively use pain medications. For side effects such as constipation, a laxative regimen can help provide the patient with relief.

Older patients often have fewer financial resources to help pay for medications, rehabilitation services, and health care assistants. They may have to go to a care facility to get services that government funding can pay for. Newer prescription plans can help defray the co-pay cost for older patients and can help these patients get the medications they need. In a recent survey of 400 nurse practitioners, respondents indicated that cost of medications was the biggest barrier to prescribing opioids for their patients (D'Arcy, 2009).

Remember: Long-term care patients have legal rights to pain relief, and elder abuse statutes have been invoked to protect older patients in pain. The most notable case of liability for undertreating pain in a patient in a nursing care facility is the case of the Estate of James vs. Hillhaven Corporation. The oncology patient had a pathologic femur fracture and had been stabilized on a medication regimen of morphine elixir. Upon admission to the nursing care facility, the nurse indicated in her assessment that the patient was receiving too much morphine and had become addicted to it. A different medication was substituted for some of the doses of morphine, and the patient died several weeks later with unrelieved pain. The patient's estate sued the facility and received $15 million in compensatory and punitive damages.

In addition to the original finding in this case, a second suit was filed by the North Carolina Department of Human Resources. As a result of this suit, the facility was fined for patient endangerment and the nurse was found liable (Pasero & McCaffrey, 2001). Other cases in different areas of the country have been filed in which undertreated pain was considered to be elder abuse (LaGanaga & Monmanney, 2001; Yi, 2001).

CHRONIC, PERSISTENT PAIN

Chronic pain, also called persistent pain, because it persists beyond the normal healing period. The following are characteristics of chronic pain:

- It lasts beyond the normal healing period.

- There may be no easily identifiable cause.

- It may be considered excessive for the degree of pathology that is identified.

- Depression is common.
  (American Pain Society, 2005; D'Arcy, 2007)

Chronic pain is very different from acute pain. Acute pain warns patients that injury has occurred and prompts them to seek medical attention to determine the source (American Pain Society, 2005). Chronic pain, on the other hand, has no real purpose but exists as a result of prior injury or undetected tissue damage. Patients with acute pain can expect to have a decrease in pain over a short period of time. For patients with chronic pain, however, there is no identifiable end point that they can use to determine when their pain will improve or resolve.

Chronic pain may have several different types of presentations, depending on the condition causing the pain:

- Pain that varies in intensity throughout the day, such as painful diabetic neuropathy (PDN), which can be more painful at night than during the day.

- Pain that increases with activity or movement, such as low back pain (LBP).

- Episodic pain that returns intermittently, such as from migraine headaches or sickle cell disease.

- Pain that is present throughout the day, such as pain from cancer or other neuropathic conditions, such as complex regional pain syndrome (CRPS), a centrally mediated pain syndrome.

For patients with chronic pain, acute pain from surgery or injury can make the chronic pain condition worse. Also, the pain from the acute source may become much more difficult to treat. The additive effect of increased pain can make the recovery process much harder for older patients, who have fewer physical and financial reserves.

PAIN CONDITIONS THAT ARE DIFFICULT TO TREAT IN OLDER PATIENTS

Some types of pain conditions that are common in older patient populations are particularly difficult to treat. This may result from the need for a multidrug medication regimen, the source of the pain (such as neuropathic pain), or the need for other forms of therapy (such as acupuncture or physical therapy). The following sections examine the more difficult-to-treat, chronic pain syndromes that affect the older patient population.

OSTEOARTHRITIS

Arthritis is a costly disease, not only in human suffering but also in financial terms. Osteoarthritis (OA) is one of the most common pain conditions that elderly patients report. The condition results from the natural aging process—weight-bearing joints lose cartilage, which produces mechanical changes, localized tissue response, and failure of function (American Pain Society, 2002). As the cartilage destruction continues, the affected bones will eventually hypertrophy (American Pain Society, 2005). More than 80% of persons over the age of 75 have OA with clinical presentation, while more than 80% of people over the age of 50 have signs of OA on radiographic studies (American Pain Society, 2002).

The joints that OA commonly affects include

- Knees

- Hips

- Feet

- Ankles

- Cervical and lower spine

- Distal interphalangeal joints

- Proximal interphalangeal joints
  (American Pain Society, 2002)

Most commonly, patients with OA report morning stiffness and pain that resolves with activity. Occasionally, patients report a "gel" phenomenon while sitting—that is, a period of stiffness that resolves in approximately 20 minutes (American Pain Society, 2002). Although activity helps resolve these stiff feelings, the pain associated with activity may make movement more difficult.

The pain of OA can be quite severe as the disease progresses and bone destruction due to hypertrophy and cartilage loss increases. More importantly, because pain limits function, activity decreases and patients can become deconditioned. This vicious cycle is self-promoting, causing more pain, less functionality, and more disability.

Depression is common for patients with OA. Because there is a high comorbidity, it is important to identify and treat depression. Patients can become socially isolated and unable to perform many of their favorite activities and pastimes. Because current therapies and treatments cannot eliminate the pain and disability of OA, it is important to consider how to treat all aspects of the condition for better treatment outcomes. Recommendations from a study with 1,800 depressed older adults found that

- Pain and depression screening should be performed for all patients with symptomatic OA.

- Use of evidence-based treatment for depression, combined with patient education and support for self-management, was effective.

- Combining treatments for pain and depression can improve treatment outcomes and decrease pain.
  (Lin et al., 2003)

Treating the pain of OA is key to retaining quality of life and functionality, and in lessening comorbidities such as depression. Recommendations for treating OA pain include

- Acetaminophen

- NSAIDs, preferably topical, or, if necessary, the lowest effective oral dose, and COX-2 medications for patients who are appropriate candidates

- Weight reduction

- Physical therapy

- Intra-articular injections with steroids, Hyalgan, or Synvisc

- Topical analgesic balms, such as capsaicin

- Physical therapy, TENS units, iontophoresis, pool-based physical therapy programs

- Arthritis Self-Management Program (ASMP)

- Joint replacements

- Opioids if pain is severe, affecting quality of life, or NSAIDs are ineffective
  (American Geriatrics Society, 2002; American Pain Society, 2002, 2005; National Institute for Health and Clinical Excellence, 2009)

Because of the chronicity of OA, combining modalities—such as medications with physical therapy, depression management, and patient education—should be considered. If the patient cannot keep up with a standard physical therapy program, using a pool-based therapy where the patient exercises in water can reduce the load on the affected joints and give the patient the feeling of successful participation in rehabilitation. A good collaborative relationship among health care professionals involved in the patient's care is essential to get the best patient outcomes and provide the patient with practical alternatives to sitting at home.

Chronic Low Back Pain

Another significant source of pain in older patients is low back pain (LBP). The pain can be classed as *axial* (low back focused), *referred* (buttock or posterior thigh), or *radicular* (radiating down the leg as a result of nerve root compression). This pain can come from any number of sources, but common causes include

- Degenerative disc disease (DDD)

- Degenerative spondylosis

- Facet syndrome

- Herniated intervertebral disc

- Spinal stenosis

- Vertebral compression fracture

  (Cayea, 2006; D'Arcy, 2009)

Approximately 6 million older adults suffer from recurrent LBP, with 36% of community-dwelling elders reporting at least one episode per year (Cayea, 2006). The problem of LBP is common, yet when surveyed, a high number of primary care practitioners indicated that they did not feel prepared to treat chronic LBP, nor did they have the knowledge of treatment options they needed (Cayea).

As with OA, LBP can be very debilitating and lead to deconditioning, social isolation, and depression. Again, screening the older patient for depression when LBP is treated can lead to a better clinical outcome and an increased quality of life.

Current recommendations by the American Pain Society (APS) and the American College of Physicians divide LBP into three categories:

- Nonspecific LBP

- Back pain potentially associated with radiculopathy or spinal stenosis

- Back pain potentially associated with another spinal cause
  (*Chou et al., 2007*)

LBP can be further divided into two major categories, acute and chronic.

- Acute LBP resolves within 6 to 12 weeks.

- Chronic LBP lasts for more than 12 weeks.

Some LBP has a radicular component, with pain running down the back of the leg, which indicates that a nerve is compressed. Other patients may complain of severe, localized pain, such as that caused by compression fractures. Each type of LBP has a particular set of symptoms that accompanies the physical deficit. Because of the variety in presentations, treatment options vary for LBP.

To treat chronic LBP, the APS low back pain guidelines (Chou et al., 2007) recommend a graduated medication schedule, coupled with additional treatments. The following medications are recommended for treating chronic LBP:

- **Acetaminophen:** The maximum daily dosage should be no more than 4,000 milligrams. If the patient uses alcohol frequently or has impaired liver function, the medication choice should be reconsidered.

- **NSAIDs:** These medications should be used at the lowest dose and the shortest possible time, but may be useful for flares, if the patient is a good candidate.

- **Opioids and tramadol:** The guidelines recommend using these medications for patients when the pain is disabling or severe after failure with acetaminophen and NSAIDS. For older patients, begin with low opioid doses. Once the patient becomes tolerant to the sedation side effect, and laxatives are used for constipation, low-dose opioids may provide enough pain relief for the patient to return to some level of activity. For older patients, tramadol may present sick serotonin syndrome, and is not fully recommended by the 2002 American Geriatrics Society Guidelines.

> **For More Information**
>
> See Chapter 3 for more information on pain medications.

Other medications that can be considered for treating chronic LBP include muscle relaxants, antidepressants (tricyclic antidepressants are *not* recommended for older patients), antiseizure medications, and herbal remedies such as capsaicin for topical use (Chou et al., 2007; Chou & Huffman, 2007; D'Arcy, 2009).

Other types of therapy that a multilevel plan of care can include are

- Acupuncture
- Exercise
- Massage
- Viniyoga-style yoga
- Progressive relaxation

- Spinal manipulation

- Interdisciplinary rehabilitation

- Transcutaneous electrical nerve stimulation (TENS)

  (Chou et al., 2007; Chou & Huffman, 2007; D'Arcy, 2009)

Since LBP pain management uses medications, it is always wise to consider what medications and what dose should be prescribed. Also, the health care provider will need to consider what medications the older patient is already taking and be aware of possible interactions with new medications. For the older patient, starting low and going slow is still a good approach to medication use, and monitoring for side effects is certainly needed when dosages are increased or new medications are added.

> **For More Information**
>
> For more information on interventional methods to control LBP, see Chapter 7.

NEUROPATHIC PAIN SYNDROMES

The International Society for the Study of Pain (IASP) defines neuropathic pain as pain that is initiated or caused by a primary lesion or dysfunction in the nervous system (peripheral or central) that disrupts impulse transmission and modulation of sensory input (Merskey & Bogduk, 1994; Polomano & Farrar, 2006). The pain can become self-perpetuating. Once pain is incorporated into a centrally mediated syndrome, such as CRPS (complex regional pain syndrome) or post-stroke pain syndrome, the ability to stop painful impulse transmission may be lost. When nervous tissue is injured or damaged, it is more difficult to treat the pain, and it is difficult to have a good outcome for pain relief. Neuropathic pain may also be caused and sustained by a continued inflammatory process. The differences in the types of pain are included in the following box.

Nociceptive Pain/Neuropathic Pain

Nociceptive Pain
- Produced in peripheral nervous system.
  - Mechanoreceptors
  - Thermoreceptors
  - Chemoreceptors
- Serves to warn the body that injury has occurred.
- Is proportionate to receptor stimulus.

Neuropathic Pain
- Caused by damage to the nervous system and continued inflammatory process and cytokine recruitment.
- Nociceptive input not required.
- Pain is of higher intensity than the injury would indicate.

For more information on the different types of pain, see Chapter 1.

Painful Diabetic Neuropathy

Neuropathic pain is a very different type of chronic pain from musculoskeletal or other nociceptive pains. One type of particularly disabling neuropathic pain is painful diabetic neuropathy (PDN). About 24 million Americans have diabetes, and many of them will develop PDN (Centers for Disease Control and Prevention, 2007). PDN usually occurs over time as a result of poorly controlled blood sugars. Patients report that they feel painful numbness in their feet; or, they may describe the sensation as feeling like they are walking on broken glass. The loss of proprioception (awareness of movement) puts the older patient at a higher risk of falls.

Assessing neuropathic pain can usually be done by listening to the descriptors a patient uses to describe the pain syndrome. When patients report the pain as burning, painful numbness; odd, painful sensations; sharp; shooting; pins and needles; or extreme sensitivity to touch, the pain should be considered neuropathic.

PDN Basics

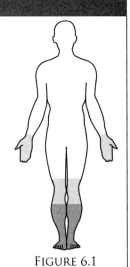

- PDN can be exacerbated by poorly controlled blood sugar levels.
- Patients report allodynia and describe the pain as sharp, stabbing, burning pain, coupled with painful numbness.
- Often presents in a stocking glove distribution (see Figure 6.1).
- Only 42% of the patients with PDN were satisfied with current treatment options.

(Dworkin et al., 2003; Weirnecke et al., 2006)

FIGURE 6.1

Treating the pain of PDN can be difficult, since many of the neuropathic pain medications cause sedation and dizziness. The older adult patient may be more sensitive to analgesic effect and need lower doses of pain medications. They may also have a higher incidence of adverse effects such as constipation (Varela-Burstein & Miller, 2003).

Recommended treatment strategies for PDN include the Stepwise Pharmacological Management Plan (Dworkin et al., 2007).

1. Assess and establish the diagnosis of neuropathic pain.

   - Establish and treat the cause of neuropathic pain.

   - Identify relevant co-morbidities.

   - Explain the diagnosis and treatment plan to the patient.

2. Treat symptoms with one or more medications.

   - Antidepressants: tricyclics (TCAs) or serotonin-norepinephrine reuptake inhibitors (SNRIs)

   - Calcium channel alpha 2 ligand drugs

- Lidocaine patch 5%

- Opioid analgesic or tramadol

3. Reassess pain and health-related quality of life.

    - If pain relief improved and no significant side effects, continue treatment.

    - If partial pain relief, add another first-line medication.

    - If no significant pain relief or inadequate pain relief, switch to another first-line medication.

4. If a trial of first- or second-line medications fails, consider third- or fourth-line medications or a referral to a pain specialist.

    (Dworkin et al., 2007)

When starting a medication regimen for neuropathic pain, the following are first-, second-, and third-line drug options.

First-line options:

- **Antidepressants:** TCAs such as amitriptyline and dual SNRIs are *not* recommended for older patients because of the increased risk of orthostatic hypotension and increased potential for falls.

- Calcium channel alpha-2 delta ligands: gabapentin and pregabalin

- Lidocaine patch 5%

Second-line options:

- **Opioid analgesics:** Decrease doses for older patients and monitor side effects carefully.

- **Tramadol:** The AGS does not recommend tramadol for older patients.

Third-line options:

- Antiepileptic medications

- Other antidepressants not mentioned previously

- Mexiletine

- NMDA (N-methyl D-aspartate) receptor agonists

- Topical capsaicin cream

Aside from medication management of the patient with PDN, the plan of care should include regular exercise, complementary methods, and regularly scheduled follow-ups. Unfortunately, for many patients complementary methods have not been shown to be entirely helpful.

Postherpetic Neuralgia

Postherpetic neuralgia (PHN) occurs most commonly in patients over 50 who have a herpes zoster (HZ) outbreak. Approximately 300,000 patients develop HZ annually (Sandy, 2005). HZ occurs most frequently in patients who are immunocompromised, are over the age of 50, and have little contact with children (Sandy; Hampton, 2005). The vesicular rash lasts approximately 2 to 4 weeks, and then scars form in the area of the eruption.

For patients who develop PHN, the area of the outbreak can become very sensitive—to the point where hyperalgesia and allodynia occur (Khaliq, Alam, & Puri, 2008). Some patients with PHN report that even the gentle pressure of wearing clothes over the area becomes extremely painful.

Risk factors for developing PHN after an HZ outbreak include the following:

- High levels of pain with the HZ outbreak

- Delayed or no antiviral treatment for the initial outbreak

- Older age, greater than 65 years of age, at onset
  (Hampton, 2005)

Patients who take antivirals at the onset of HZ have a 20% chance of developing PHN. For patients who do not have antiviral treatment, the rate of PHN rises to 40% (Hampton, 2005).

The following are treatment options for PHN:

- Recommended

    - Tricyclic antidepressants (Staats et al., 2004)

    - Gabapentin, pregabalin (Staats et al., 2004)

    - Opioids

    - Topical lidocaine patches 5% (Davies & Galer, 2004)

- Low benefit

    - Aspirin cream

    - Capsaicin cream

- Insufficient evidence or no benefit

    - Acupuncture

    - Dorsal root, or stellate ganglion blocks

    - Dextromethorphan, indomethacin, epidural morphine sulfate, epidural methylprednisolone, carbemazapine, ketamine, lorazepam, vitamin E

  (Morantz & Torrey, 2005)

Older patients who are at risk for developing HZ should be vaccinated for HZ. Findings indicate that patients who get HZ after receiving the vaccination develop a less severe form of the illness when it does occur, and fewer vaccinated patients develop PHN (Oxman et al., 2005).

Post-Treatment Neuropathies, Chemotherapy-Related Neuropathy, and Post-Mastectomy/Post-Thoracotomy Pain Syndromes

In some instances, surgery and therapies designed to treat disease create a post-treatment pain condition that is neuropathic. Approximately 20% of women who have a mastectomy or lumpectomy for cancer develop a neuropathic pain condition called *postmastectomy pain* (Polomano & Farrar, 2006). This syndrome is more common in younger women and those who are overweight. Often, patients with this syndrome will complain of "strange sensations" in the surgical axilla or painful numbness, pins and needles, or burning sensation. Treatment for this condition follows the stepwise recommendations listed previously.

Patients who receive vinca alkaloid, taxanes, platinum-based compounds, cytosine arabinoside, fluorouracil, and animitotic agents can develop a condition called *chemotherapy-related neuropathy*. The condition develops in a stocking glove distribution and can develop very quickly or take months to develop (Polomano & Farrar, 2006). The condition can be dose-related. Decreasing dosing regimens, if possible, once symptoms develop can potentially decrease the progress of the neuropathy.

Post-thoracotomy pain syndrome (PTPS) occurs in approximately 50% to 80% of patients who undergo thoracotomy (Polomano & Farrar, 2006). Approximately 5% of patients who develop PTPS experience long-term, debilitating pain. Patients have described this pain as being like a blow torch covering the chest wall area. The origin of the pain is thought to be damage to the intercostal nerves during surgery (Wallace & Wallace, 1997).

Other chronic illnesses and post-treatment syndromes occur with some regularity. Phantom limb pain occurs in 30% to 81% of all patients who have a lower limb amputated (Eichenberger et al., 2008). HIV neuropathy occurs in patients with HIV disease. The common complaints with HIV neuropathy are allodynia and hyperalgesia (Abrams et al., 2007). Finally, complex regional pain syndrome (CRPS) can occur as a result of a crush injury or from inadequately managed postoperative pain (D'Arcy, 2007).

Regardless of the cause, the conditions are extremely painful and difficult to treat. For the older patient, developing a condition such as PHN can put an end to independent living, destroy quality of life, and cause depression and social isolation. Treating chronic, persistent pain in older adults can provide the support the individual needs to continue living with a good, productive quality of life.

Treating Pain in Long-Term Care

According to American Health Care Association (AHCA) nursing home statistics (n.d.), between 1.5 and 1.6 million frail elderly patients live in long-term care facilities. These facilities include nursing homes, skilled nursing facilities, rehabilitation facilities, and other facilities where the patient resides and can receive help with care on a daily basis. Many of the patients are the elite elderly, age 85 and over, who comprise the oldest group of patients; those with medical conditions that are difficult to handle at home; and patients with terminal illnesses such as cancer. Many have dementia or are cognitively impaired in some way, and have been institutionalized for long periods of time.

Despite being a vulnerable population, these older patients are some of the most overlooked and undertreated patients with pain. There are significant difficulties with assessing pain in this group of patients. Getting an accurate report of pain can be a challenge, even with older patients who are verbal and mentally intact. Simple, easy-to-use scales are best, and ensuring that assistive devices are in use can help make the communication about pain easier. Residents of long-term facilities seem to prefer the verbal descriptor scale, with simple word cues, or the FACES scale (Hutt, Buffum, Fink, Jones, & Pepper, 2007).

The nonverbal patient presents a completely different challenge, since behavioral pain scales must be used to assess pain. Some of these behavioral changes are very subtle and may represent other comorbidities, such as depression, or other conditions such as thirst or hunger (Hutt et al., 2007). For patients who are assessed for pain using an observational tool, using one intervention at a time may help determine if the behaviors are truly representative of pain (Hutt et al.).

At first glance, these patients seem to be the most difficult to treat with medication, because they are sensitive to opioids and have physiologic changes, such as decreased liver and kidney functions. Because they are perceived as difficult to treat, these patients are easily overlooked and undertreated. In a study by Huffman and Kunik (2000) of 97 institutionalized older patients, 66% had pain, but only 15% had received any analgesics in the last 24 hours. A number of pain medications can be used with this population, but reducing dosages and using the "start low, go slow" concept are the best approaches.

DEMENTIA AND PAIN

The prevalence of dementia in patients older than 65 years of age is higher in women than men (Matthews & Dening, 2002). In a UK study of 13,004 older people (those over the age of 65) 5% lived in institutions, and prevalence of dementia within the institutionalized older patients was 62% (Matthews & Dening). Studies by the AGS (2002) showed that 45% to 80% of all patients in long-term care had chronic, daily pain.

For patients with dementia, pain sensitization and the sensory component of pain seem to be intact (Huffman & Kunik, 2000). Individuals with dementia seem to be able to localize pain stimulus and activate a basic withdrawal reaction to the pain. They also appear to have an intact pain threshold and the ability to discriminate pain intensity by increasing response or hyper-reactivity to pain (Huffman & Kunik). Interestingly, since the amygdala atrophies with dementia and can have amyloid plaquing at varying levels, the pain response may be different depending on the amount of physiologic changes that have taken place (Huffman & Kunik).

In patients with dementia, the affective response to pain is different. The patient's body may be able to experience the pain stimulus, but the individual may be unable to identify the experience as pain and interpret the meaning of the pain.

The physiologic changes mean that, to some extent, pain can be processed in cognitively impaired and demented individuals; however, there seems to be a decreased rate of pain complaints in this patient population. In a group of older patients receiving lumbar punctures, patients with dementia had a 2% decrease in post-lumbar puncture headache, and the incidence of the headache decreased with the severity of the dementia (Huffman & Kunik, 2000). When a group of demented patients and another group of cognitively intact patients were assessed for the top 25 symptoms of older patients, the demented group had significantly fewer complaints of pain in five of the pain-related symptoms, with less joint pain being a significant finding (Huffman & Kunik).

Thus, although the prevalence of pain in these vulnerable individuals is high, pain complaints may be decreased when compared to those of cognitively intact elders. The assessment process and inability to self-report pain seem to be integral to this gap. Memory loss can impact the abilities both to communicate and to recall the meaning of prior painful sensations (Buffum, Miaskowski, & Sands, 2001). When a health care provider is assessing a demented or cognitively impaired patient, the following behaviors can be helpful in determining whether the patient is in pain:

- Agitation

- Pacing

- Verbal aggression

- Grimacing

- Frowning

- Tense body posture

- Fidgeting

- Wandering

- Noisy breathing
  (Buffum et al., 2001)

CONSIDERATIONS FOR TREATING PAIN IN LONG-TERM CARE

Once behaviors in nonverbal patients are identified as pain-related or suspected to be pain-related, an analgesic trial may prove effective if the behaviors decrease with the medication. Recommendations for treating pain in nonverbal patients include:

- Using scheduled medication administration rather than providing medication "as needed."

- Encouraging patients who are able to request pain medication to do so when in pain. In a study of 2,033 nursing home residents, 53% admitted to being in pain, and 60% of those patients had not requested anything for pain (Hutt et al., 2007).

- Using an extended release medication to provide consistent pain relief for patients who have been using regular pain medication.

- Identifying the type of pain the patient is experiencing. Neuropathic pain will require a medication regimen that includes a medication designed for neuropathic pain.

- Matching the type of medication with the severity of the pain. That is, for mild pain, use nonopioids; for moderate pain, use weaker compound opioids; and for severe pain, use strong opioids (Hutt et al., 2007). See Chapter 3 for more detailed information.

- Addressing side effects such as constipation, sedation, impaired cognition and balance, and gastrointestinal bleeding.
  (Hutt et al., 2007)

Finally, to treat pain successfully in the long-term care patient population, assessment for pain and side effects should be a continuous process. When opioids are started, frequent reassessment must take place to ensure that patients can tolerate the medication and dose, and that side effects are not occurring. Consider adding nonpharmacologic therapies to augment pain relief from medications.

For More Information

For more information about nonpharmacologic therapies, see Chapter 4.

Summary

The older patient can have a wide variety of chronic pain conditions. Helping to decrease pain can lead to increased functionality and a higher quality of life. Some older patients are difficult to assess because of communication barriers, such as aphasia after a stroke or dementia. Learning to assess the patient who cannot self-report pain can help decrease the amount of pain and improve quality of life. It is also important to determine the type of pain—nociceptive or neuropathic—to ensure that the correct medication is used to decrease the pain.

Chronic pain may be prevalent in the older patient, but that does not mean it cannot be treated. Using medications, interventional techniques, and integrative therapies can provide the older patients with adequate pain relief and ensure the best outcomes possible.

CASE STUDY

Jim James is a 77-year-old man who has a long history of low back pain related to a work injury in his younger years. Last year, he had herpes zoster (HZ), which resulted in residual pain over his chest wall. He likes to fish and garden, but last summer he was unable to do so because of the new HZ pain. A widower, he lives by himself but has three children nearby. His children think Jim should give up his home and live with one of them, but he prefers to stay in his own home.

When Jim comes to see you about his continuing pain, he says, "The pain just does not stop. I was pretty much able to do what I wanted before the HZ, if I took my pain medicine. I couldn't do heavy lifting, but I could fish and garden and see my kids and grandkids. Now I am pretty much confined to a chair watching ballgames. I don't sleep very well, and I have to agree with my daughter, who says my house could use a good cleaning. What can you do to help my pain, so I can get my life back?"

You perform a history and physical and find that Jim has pronounced hypersensitivity to normal touch in the area of the healed HZ lesions. He has low back pain that does not radiate. His pain rating for the HZ is 6/10 and for his back pain, 5/10. His Neuropathic Pain Scale score is in the high range. He describes the pain as a constant burning sensation in his chest wall. He appears fatigued and depressed and reports he is constipated.

In the past, Jim had been using one or two oxycodone/APAP tablets a day, and his activity had decreased the back pain. Sitting all day has exacerbated his back pain. Now he is taking 20 mg of extended release oxycodone a day and six tablets of oxycodone/APAP for breakthrough pain, but he still has severe pain.

Critical Analysis Questions

1. In older patients, drugs can remain longer in the tissues because older patients have decreased lean body mass, increased body fat, decreased total body water, and increased plasma protein. Lipid solubility and protein binding are directly affected by these changes. How will this affect the choice of medications for Jim's pain?

2. What type of condition is Jim's HZ pain called?

3. What types of medications would you consider effective for Jim's pain?

   - More or different opioids
   - Lidocaine patch
   - Antidepressants
   - Antiepileptic medications
   - Capsaicin cream
   - NSAIDs
   - Other

4. How would you address Jim's depression? What elements of his condition contribute to his feeling depressed? Does he need a referral to a psychiatrist?

5. Is Jim addicted to or dependent on his opioids?

7

INTERVENTIONAL PAIN MANAGEMENT FOR OLDER PATIENTS

For certain painful conditions that affect older patients, such as low back pain or neuropathic pain, interventional pain management is an appropriate choice. Interventional pain-management techniques can either be used alone or as part of the treatment regimen, depending on the type of pain and the needs of the patient. These techniques can provide pain relief while reducing or eliminating the use of oral medications, and many are performed on an out-patient basis—thus no hospital stay is involved. Pain relief can be almost immediate, as with vertebroplasty, or take days or weeks to develop, as with spinal injections.

The following are some of the more common interventional pain management techniques:

- Nerve blocks such as epidural steroid injections, selective nerve blocks, and facet injections

- Spinal cord stimulation

- Implanted intrathecal pumps

- Vertebroplasty and kyphoplasty

To obtain a specialized injection or treatment, patients usually must be referred to a pain management specialist, orthopedist, acupuncturist, or neurosurgeon. The following questions should be considered when determining whether a patient referral is indicated:

- Does the patient have uncontrolled, severe pain that has not been responsive to the usual medications and dose titrations?

- Is there a comorbid psychiatric condition, such as depression, anxiety, or alcohol or substance abuse?

- Does the patient have declining physical condition or deteriorating coping skills?

- Is a referral needed to make or confirm a diagnosis?

- Would a referral be helpful in obtaining treatment recommendations for specific pain complaints?

- Would the referral provide treatment options that the current primary care practitioner cannot provide?

(APS, 2006)

Discussion about alcohol use should take place even with older adult patients. Alcohol use might seem less likely in this population, but many older adults use alcohol to ease pain and discomfort, since it does not require a visit to a physician or a prescription, and it is easily available. The use of alcohol in an older patient may be an indication of undertreated pain that could be resolved by changing medications or doses or by interventional pain management.

> **For More Information**
>
> Additional interventional pain management techniques include acupuncture (see Chapter 4) and intra-articular injections (see Chapter 6).

ACUPUNCTURE

As mentioned in Chapter 4, acupuncture uses thin needles, inserted into designated areas of the body, to channel energy into blocked areas to improve circulation and flow. Originally a Chinese therapy, acupuncture has now found favor worldwide. The treatment is as effective as the practitioner's skills permit, so patients considering acupuncture for pain relief should conduct a thorough review of the qualifications of the practitioner.

To study the efficacy of acupuncture, a meta-analysis (Manheimer, White, Berman, Forys, & Ernst, 2005) analyzed results from sham acupuncture sessions versus real acupuncture treatment. Research findings indicate that acupuncture is a good option for treatment of chronic low back pain. The data for acute low back pain is not conclusive, and therefore no recommendation was made for that type of pain (Manheimer et al.).

INTERVENTIONAL MODALITIES FOR PAIN MANAGEMENT

As patients age, arthritis and other conditions can change the normal (see Figure 7.1) individual spinal processes, creating

- bone spurs that can compress soft tissue or nerves

- facet arthropathy that impinges on nerve roots

- disc desiccation and degenerative disc disease (DDD), which cause pressure on spinal nerves as the cushioning between vertebrae thins

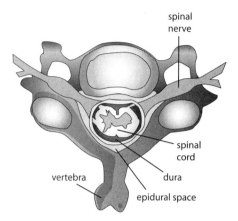

FIGURE 7.1   CROSS-SECTION OF NORMAL SPINAL PROCESSES

In other cases, patients who have back surgery that fails to relieve the original pain complaint have what is called *failed back syndrome*. Other patients have a back injury that results in a herniated nucleus pulposus (HNP), which can press on the adjacent nerve root, causing pain. Some of these patients develop radicular pain that radiates down one or both legs. Patients may call this condition *sciatica* or *radiculopathy*.

The spinal bones can thicken with age and create internal pressure on the spinal cord, creating *spinal stenosis* that is extremely painful and limits mobility. Patients with spinal stenosis will eventually develop a stooped posture with a widened gait. These problems can be treated with interventional options, if the patient is willing (and able) to undergo a procedure and the insurance company agrees to pay for the cost.

The more common interventional options for pain relief consist of an injection at a nerve root or spinal facet with a preservative-free combination of steroids and local anesthetics to reduce inflammation and provide analgesia. Less commonly, a procedure that affects nerve roots, such as *radiofrequency lesioning*, or specific muscle groups, such as *prolotherapy*, may be used.

Because these techniques are newer in the pain management discipline, limited research is available; as a result, support may not be strong for these techniques. This does not mean the techniques have no value, just that the literature to provide research support may be too sparse. A Cochrane review (Nelemans, deBie, deVet, & Sturmans, 2000) reported no convincing evidence for the effect of injection therapy on subacute or chronic low back pain. In a systematic review of findings, injection therapy was not shown to be more effective than placebo (Nelemans et al.). Research supporting the American Pain Society's guidelines on low back pain had similar findings (Chou & Huffman, 2007). However, anecdotally, many patients seem to benefit from the technique.

For most of the injection techniques, the medication is placed directly at the source or site of the pain.

- **Steroid injections:** Epidural steroid injection (ESI) can be performed in the cervical, thoracic, lumbar, and caudal epidural space. A solution of preservative-free steroid, such as depomedrol, is combined with a local anesthetic, such as bupivacaine or ropivacaine, and then injected at the level of the nerve creating the pain. This provides localized relief directly at the source of the pain (Armon, Argoff, Samuels, & Backonja, 2007).

  Preauthorization from the insurance provider is needed, and insurance usually covers the initial assessment and two injections. A series of three injections in a 12-month period is the maximum number that most pain specialists will perform, so the last injection may require a reauthorization. Patients can usually expect the pain to decrease slowly over 5 to 7 days if the injection is effective. Even with the use of fluoroscopy, there is no guarantee that the medication can be placed directly into the area of the nerve root. This means that some patients may have no relief or only partial relief, but subsequent injections may provide an increase in pain relief as the effect spreads.

- **Trigger point injections:** Typically performed when a patient can identify a specific spot on their body that is painful. Local anesthetic (lidocaine) is injected directly into the painful area.

Although not heavily supported by research, trigger point injections are often used for patients who have tender points with fibromyalgia.

- **Prolotherapy:** This treatment involves injections of an irritant solution into weakened back muscles, which stimulates an inflammatory response and a reduction in muscle laxity. It does not have enough research evidence to support using it alone. However, when this technique is combined with a structured physical therapy regimen aimed at rehabilitation, the injections are more beneficial than control injections (Dagenais, Yelland, Del Ma, & Schoene, 2009).

- **Radiofrequency lesioning, intradiscal electrothermal therapy (IDET):** Using a heated probe to transect the nerve in the painful area has found support in some practices. This practice has provided anecdotal reports of relief for discogenic back pain. However, in a randomized, double-blind, controlled trial of IDET versus placebo, the findings revealed no significant benefit for the treated patients over the placebo group (Freeman, Fraser, Cain, Hall, & Chappie, 2005).

- **Epiduroscopy:** The insertion of a scope into the epidural space to use specialized tools to remove scar tissue from nerve roots has been trialed with limited success. There is insufficient research to indicate if the risk-to-benefit ratio of this technique merits its use.

Implanted Modalities

When pain management reaches a point where manipulating medications and simple interventional options such as epidural spinal injections do not provide adequate pain relief, an implanted modality may be considered. These modalities include intrathecal implanted pumps and spinal cord stimulators. While spinal cord stimulators are designed to treat neuropathic pain syndromes, intrathecal pumps can be used to treat the pain of low back pain syndromes and other chronic and oncology pain conditions.

IMPLANTED INTRATHECAL PUMPS

Intrathecal drug delivery systems are used to control chronic pain in patients who have exhausted all other medication management and have maximized medication doses. Before considering this type of therapy, patients should have had an extended trial of various medications, medication doses, and combinations of treatments and medications.

Intrathecal drug delivery consists of an implanted computerized pump that automatically delivers a prescribed dose of medication at a set rate. The medication is delivered from the pump into the intrathecal space via a flexible catheter that is tunneled from the spinal insertion point along the lateral aspect of the patient's body, and then connected to the pump. The pump is secured by surgically inserting it into a pocket in the abdominal or other subcutaneous tissue close to the skin's surface. The pump is kept close to the skin to make refilling the pump easier. How soon refilling is needed is determined by the pump volume, medication concentration, and the infusion rate of the medication. Higher rates require more frequent refills. A special refill kit is used to access the pump reservoir's port to withdraw any leftover medication and inject the new medication. The pump refill date is then reset to a new date that is determined by the concentration of the medication and medication delivery rate.

The following medications are approved by the FDA for use in implanted intrathecal pumps:

- Morphine

- Baclofen (Lioresal)

- Ziconotide (Prialt)

Medications used in implanted intrathecal pumps should be preservative-free. Morphine is the most common medication, and using an intrathecal medication delivery system can provide doses that are 300 times as potent as oral morphine (Wallace & Staats, 2005). Before the pump is permanently implanted, a trial should be performed using an external intrathecal or epidural catheter, and the anticipated medication, generally morphine. During the trial period, the drug selection is based on the following:

- History of opioid tolerance

- History of side effects

- Pain-afferent spinal cord level, compared with catheter tip location

  (Wallace & Staats, 2005)

The lipophilicity of the selected pain medication and the available lipid supply of the spinal cord, as well as the accessibility of the cerebrospinal fluid and blood supply, can directly affect the analgesic action of the medication being used (Wallace & Staats, 2005).

Ziconotide is a one-of-a-kind medication, classed as a neuronal-type (N-type) calcium channel blocker. Derived from the venom of the cone snail, a marine variety, Ziconotide must be administered intrathecally using a continuous infusion (Lynch, Cheng, & Yee, 2006). It can be used to treat both chronic nociceptive and neuropathic pain (Schroeder, Doering, Zamponi, & Lewis, 2006). The following side effects, mainly neuropsychiatric, can be significant:

> **Clinical Tip**
>
> Ziconotide should be reserved for patients who have failed all other, more conventional, medications and interventions.

- Depression

- Cognitive impairment

- Depressed levels of consciousness

- Hallucinations

- Elevated creatine kinase levels

  (Lynch et al., 2006)

Practitioners are using other medications in implanted pumps when pain is not controlled with standard medication, but the risk of pump malfunction increases when unapproved medications are used.

Clinical Tip

The idea of implanting a foreign device that will deliver pain medication with no or limited ability for the patient to control it can be an unsettling decision. For the technique to be successful, a careful evaluation of the candidate prior to implantation is essential. The criteria for selecting a candidate for intrathecal medication delivery include:

- Ineffective oral analgesia with multiple oral or transcutaneous trials, including dose titration.
- Intolerable side effects, despite opioid rotation.
- Functional analgesia during temporary trial infusion.
- Psychologic stability and reasonable goals.
- Access to care—the patient will return to the pain clinic for pump refills and dose adjustments.
- Patient acceptance.
- For baclofen—intractable spasticity unrelieved by oral antispasmodics, with improved spasticity with baclofen test dosing.

(Wallace & Staats, 2005)

The use of an intrathecal medication delivery system can have a number of problems. The patient risk-benefit ratio should be weighed carefully; all other reasonable options should be tried before pump implantation. If the patient does not have a 50% reduction in pain levels with the pre-pump implantation trial, the final implantation should be reconsidered.

Before the catheter is placed, the patient should be aware of certain risks. Consider the following when administering intrathecal medications:

- Catheter placement can be difficult if the patient has spinal deformity, prior spinal surgery, or abdominal surgery.

- Patients are at risk for infection, meningitis, arachnoiditis, and catheter-related granuloma formation.

- Anticoagulation can cause a compressive hematoma when the catheter is being placed or removed.

- A pump malfunction can cause a withdrawal syndrome.

- Intrathecal medications can cause low-pressure spinal headaches.

- Tolerance can develop, which may result in escalation of dose.
  (Wallace & Staats, 2005)

Spinal Cord Stimulation

Although the mechanism of spinal cord stimulation (SCS) is poorly understood at this time, it is best characterized as a technique that represents the gate control theory of pain relief. In the gate control theory, repeated painful stimuli open the gate for pain transmission. SCS can selectively depolarize large fiber afferents in the dorsal columns of the spinal cord, thereby closing the gate without causing motor effect (Wallace & Staats, 2005). The pulse generation of the stimulator may activate the sympathetic nervous system. Other neuronal pathways may also be activated, providing additional pain relief (Wallace & Staats).

Clinical Tip

Consider the following criteria when selecting patients for SCS:
- All acceptable and less invasive treatment options should be exhausted.
- Patients should be evaluated for any psychiatric comorbidities, issues of substance abuse, and potential for secondary gain.
- A diagnosis should be established for the pain.
- SCS should be limited to patients who received a good level of pain relief and functional improvement during test stimulation trials.

(Adapted from Wallace & Staats, 2005; Neuromodulation Therapy Access Coalition [NTAC], 2008)

Simplistically, the device consists of an implanted generator that delivers electrical pulses to a lead located in the targeted spinal cord area that is thought to be the pain source (Mailis-Gagnon, Furlan, Sandoval, & Taylor, 2008). The generator is attached to a lead (or leads) implanted in the epidural space at the site of pain generation, either percutaneously or through a laminectomy. When the system is activated, the patient will feel tingling, or paresthesia, over the affected or painful area. Patients who are considering this type of pain relief modality should be aware that it might take several trials and lead manipulations to find the best combination for pain relief.

SCS is considered to be a useful form of pain relief for patients with the following conditions:

- Failed back syndrome, with pain continuing despite operative procedures to relieve the source of the pain

- Chronic, intractable pain of the trunk or limbs

- Chronic, neuropathic pain; complex regional pain syndrome (CRPS); phantom pain; painful diabetic neuropathy (PDN); and post-herpetic neuralgia (PHN)

  (Mailis-Gagnon et al., 2008; NTAC, 2008)

The clinician should give patients being considered for SCS a very thorough physical and psychological examination. Older patients should also be tested to see if they understand the technique well enough to manage the handheld programmer, which turns the stimulator off and on and adjusts stimulation levels. Before using SCS, patients should have tried medication management and different combinations and doses of medication with limited results. Although research results are mixed and limited, the technique is a treatment option covered by Medicare and other governmental health care programs, all major commercial health plans, and most workers compensation plans in the United States (NTAC, 2008). The chance that SCS will work and increase function is an outcome that should be considered if the trial stimulation relieves pain. The last positive aspect of SCS is that it is minimally invasive, reversible, and nondestructive; if the technique does not provide the expected result, the lead(s) and generator can be removed (NTAC).

> ## Clinical Tip
>
> Contraindications for SCS are as follows:
> - Coagulopathy
> - Sepsis
> - Untreated major co-morbidity, such as depression
> - Serious drug or behavior problem
> - Inability to operate or control the device
> - Secondary gain
> - On-demand cardiac pacemaker
>
> (Wallace & Staats, 2005)

The clinician should attempt medication and dose adjustment before considering an implanted modality to treat a patient's pain. Once the patient receives an implanted device, the pain clinic practitioner and patient are closely linked, and frequent pain clinic visits are required. For older patients who have difficulty finding transportation to a clinic, another pain relief option should be considered.

Osteoporotic Compression Fractures

Osteoporosis is a disorder that causes bones to lose density and become porous and fragile (Smeltzer, 2007). A common disorder in older, postmenopausal women, it contributes to compression fractures that can be incredibly painful. Osteoporosis affects more women than men because after menopause, women have decreased estrogen levels, which cause increased bone resorption (Smeltzer). Osteoporotic spinal bones are more fragile and porous than normal bone (see Figure 7.2), which results in an increased risk of vertebral compression fracture and compression of spinal nerve roots.

Although osteoporosis itself is not painful, the resulting compression fractures can result in restricted functional ability and a need for opioids, which can lead to adverse events such as sedation, constipation, and nausea.

When a patient develops osteoporosis, the bones not only lose density and appear moth-eaten and porous, but they also lose structure. The patient loses bone faster than it is created, resulting in spinal deformities and loss of vertebral height as the vertebrae collapse. The vertebral fracture and collapse result in progressive kyphosis and height loss (Figure 7.3). This progressive forward position tends to force the spine into a rounded, kyphotic curve, while the head is pushed forward into a downward-looking position.

The changes in bone density and bone fragility are significant for a number of reasons. A kyphotic posture can be a safety risk and cause falls that result in spinal fractures, and pain and disability associated with compression fractures can lead to significant deconditioning in an older patient.

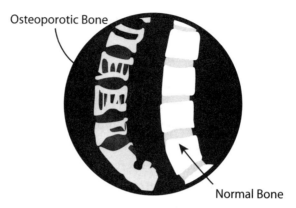

Osteoporotic Bone

Normal Bone

© http://hpb.gov.sg/data/hpb.home/files/pro/strongbonesforlife_e_.pdf

Figure 7.2   Comparison of osteoporotic and normal bone

More than 100 million people worldwide, 44 million in the United States, are estimated to be at risk for developing vertebral fractures related to osteoporosis (Phillips, 2003). Approximately 700,000 spinal fractures occur each year in the United States, one-third of which become chronically painful (Hulme, Krebs, Ferguson, & Berlemann, 2006; Phillips). Every year, the pain and subsequent disability from these fractures result in more than 800,000 emergency department visits, more than 2.6 million outpatient visits, and more than 180,000 older adults being placed in long-term care facilities (Smeltzer, 2007).

Some patients can tell when the fracture occurs. For many the cause of the fracture may be a simple motion, such as lifting plates down from a shelf. For others, a sudden trip or fall may result in a compression fracture. Yet other patients will state that they have no idea what caused the fracture; they may simply wake up one morning with severe back pain. The pain of the fracture can be severe, regardless of the cause. As the vertebrae collapse and nerves are entrapped or compressed, the pain can become intense and debilitating.

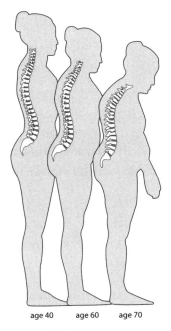

age 40   age 60   age 70

Progression of Vertebral Fractures in Osteoporosis

FIGURE 7.3   KYPHOSIS FROM OSTEOPOROSIS

The patient who is experiencing pain from a compression fracture may report a severe level of pain, 7/10 to 10/10, at a specific site on his or her back. Unfortunately, because some of the pain is caused by nerve root impingement, the normal medications for pain are less than effective and can have unwanted side effects such as sedation, confusion, and nausea and vomiting. Even though the common compression fracture is found in older patients, opioids are often used because the pain intensity is reported as being severe. This can lead to sedation, nausea, and, if continued, constipation. Other treatment options provide excellent pain relief in a very short period of time, but they require a procedure such as vertebroplasty or kyphoplasty. Health care providers who work with older patients on a regular basis should consider what may contribute to osteoporosis and look for ways of treating the condition to reduce the risk of compression fracture.

Determining Risk for Osteoporosis

When evaluating a patient's risk for osteoporosis, it is important to review his or her lifestyle habits and medications.

The following lifestyle practices, medical conditions, and medications are known to reduce calcium deposition and retention in bones:

- The use of caffeine, alcohol, and carbonated soft drinks; a sedentary lifestyle; and low calcium intake (all of which can lead to *primary osteoporosis*)

- Celiac disease, hypogonadism, lactose intolerance, hyperthyroidism, renal and liver failure, and anorexia (all of which can lead to *secondary osteoporosis*)

- Corticosteroids, antiseizure medications, heparin, tetracycline, aluminum-containing antacids, and thyroid supplements
  (Smeltzer, 2007)

Patients who are high risk may take a medication designed to increase calcium deposition and retention. These medications include

- Bisphosphonates such as alendronate (Fosamax)

- Risedronate (Actonel)

- Ibandronate (Boniva)

- Zoledronic acid (Reclast)
  (National Institutes of Health [NIH], 2008)

This type of medication can have significant side effects, such as gastrointestinal problems—difficulty swallowing, inflammation of the esophagus, and gastric ulcer (NIH, n.d.). Estrogen receptor modulators such as raloxifene (Evista), estrogen replacement therapy (a controversial treatment option), and calcitonin (a hormone used to regulate calcium) are also used to treat osteoporosis (NIH).

Patients who complain of back pain and are at risk for decreased bone density because of lifestyle factors, comorbidities, or medication use should be screened for compression fractures. Patients who have had a compression fracture are at a much higher risk for repeat fracture. A standard spinal MRI can reveal the extent of the spinal compression and any vertebral fractures. Bone density scans can also be helpful in determining how to adjust medication to improve calcium absorption and retention.

PATIENT EDUCATION RELATED TO RISK FACTORS

Patient education for high-risk patients, such as Caucasian women with small frames, should be provided to help minimize the effects of osteoporosis. For example, some patients might not be taking the right amount of calcium. Patients 19 to 50 years of age should take 1,000mg per day, and adults over 50 should take 1,200mg. Calcium supplements often include 400 to 600IU of vitamin D, which is necessary for calcium absorption (Smeltzer, 2007). Patients should also be taught the adverse events that can occur with vitamin supplementation, such as kidney stones and vitamin D toxicity.

Regular exercise, including resistance and impact exercise, is encouraged to help to create bone mass and retain structure. Patients should also be discouraged from smoking and from regular use of alcohol, caffeine, and carbonated beverages.

CONSIDERING TREATMENT OPTIONS

Teriperatide (Forteo) is a parathyroid compound approved for treating postmenopausal women who are at high risk for fracture (Kessenich, 2003). Although medication approach is not new, the results of a randomized clinical trial with a cohort of 1,637 women found that subcutaneous injections of 800 units of parathyroid hormone (PTH) decreased risk of vertebral fracture and increased bone density

(Kessenich). For women who have had a compression fracture, any treatment that can help maintain the remaining bone structures and retain calcium should be considered. Adherence with treatment is very important; the continued use of PTH is the only way to retain the benefit (Barclay & Lie, 2008; Prince, Devine, Sarvinder, & Dick, 2006).

Medications such as opioids, nonsteroidal inflammatory drugs (NSAIDs), and topical agents such as analgesic balms are options for treating the pain of compression fractures. Adverse side effects such as sedation, constipation, confusion, or comorbid cardiovascular disease can limit use of opioids. Bedrest and braces can also decrease pain. In addition, some new interventional methods have been found to be extremely helpful and successful for relieving the pain of compression fractures.

Interventional Options for Relieving the Pain of Compression Fractures

Vertebroplasty and kyphoplasty are two minimally invasive interventional techniques that can be performed as outpatient procedures. These procedures can dramatically reduce the pain of the fracture in a short period of time.

Vertebroplasty was first introduced in 1987 to treat the pain of vertebral fractures (Hulme et al., 2006). To perform the procedure, a polyacrylic cement is inserted into the deformed vertebra to help stabilize the fractures or decrease the kyphotic angle of the vertebra (see Figure 7.4).

Kyphoplasty was first used in 1998 to help realign spinal deformities and increase the height of the vertebral body (Hulme et al., 2006). A somewhat more detailed procedure than vertebroplasty, kyphoplasty involves the percutaneous injection of PMMA into a space created by a bone tamp that has an inflatable balloon (Hulme et al., 2006, Figure 7.5). Filling the new space with the cement medium can help to correct the kyphotic angle of the spine and reduce the potential for new fractures.

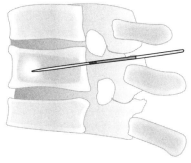

FIGURE 7.4   VERTEBROPLASTY

A biopsy needle is guided into the fractured vertebra through a small skin incision. Acrylic bone cement is shown flowing into the vertebra, filling the spaces within the bone. The restored vertebra stabilizes the vertebral structure and relieves the pain.

Vertebroplasty/Kyphoplasty

Vertebroplasty

Vertebroplasty is the percutaneous injection of polymethylmethacrylate (PMMA) directly into the fractured vertebral body (Phillips, 2003).

Kyphoplasty

Kyphoplasty is the percutaneous injection of PMMA in a cavity created in the vertebra that, when filled, will help correct the kyphotic angle of the spine (Phillips, 2003).

The value of these techniques is the quick recovery and pain relief provided once the procedure is completed. Almost all patients can have a vertebroplasty or kyphoplasty as an outpatient and return home the same day.

In a systematic review of 69 clinical studies using either vertebroplasty or kyphoplasty with 2,958 patients, 87% of the vertebroplasty patients and 92% of the kyphoplasty patients had pain relief (Hulme et al., 2006). Visual analog pain scale ratings were reduced from 8.2 on a 0 to 10 scale to 3.0 for vertebroplasty and from 7.4 to 3.4 for kyphoplasty (Hulme et al.). Given the severity of the pre-procedure pain and the limited efficacy of the conservative measures, the pain relief from these minimally invasive procedures is dramatic.

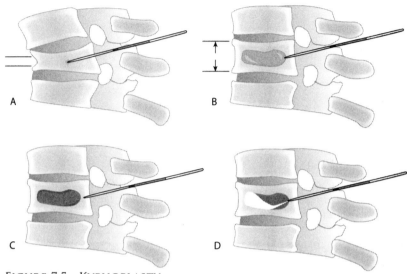

FIGURE 7.5   KYPHOPLASTY

A, Percutaneous cannulation of the fractured vertebral body with placement of the inflatable bone tamp (IBT). B, IBT inflation elevating the vertebral body end plates and restoring vertebral body height. C, IBT is withdrawn leaving a cavity to be filled with bone void filler. D, Bone void filler is placed into the vertebral body under low pressure.

Complications, though infrequent, can be associated with the two procedures, including

- Infection

- Fractures of the transverse process, pedicle, sternum, and ribs

- Respiratory distress as result of anesthesia

- Cement leakage (occurred in 41% of vertebroplasties in the review studies and 9% of the kyphoplasties)

    (Hulme et al., 2006)

SUMMARY

Interventional pain management options are appropriate for selected patients. For those patients who do not get adequate pain relief with medication management and dose adjustments, choosing an interventional option such as steroid injections can provide added pain relief that can improve the quality of life and functionality of the patients. Although not all interventional treatments have sufficient evidence to support them, the positive clinical outcomes seem to support their use in clinical practice if indicated for the patient. These techniques are evolving, and as they progress, more information will be available for patients and health care providers to weigh the risks and benefits for all interventional options.

CASE STUDY

James Jones is an 82-year-old man with a long history of chronic low back pain. He lives with his elderly wife, who is quite debilitated with arthritis and depends on Mr. Jones to do her shopping and some of the house care.

Mr. Jones first hurt his back in a motor vehicle accident when he was in his 40s. At that time, he had several different surgeries in an attempt to restore function and regain his former lifestyle. Despite the best efforts of the surgeon, Mr. Jones was left with intractable pain that ranged from 3/10 at the very best to 8/10 with flares. During the last 40 years, Mr. Jones has taken many different medications and tried various techniques for pain relief. Nothing seems to work all the time. He is currently on a fentanyl patch, 75mcg/h strength, and uses acetaminophen and oxycodone (Percocet) for breakthrough pain. He cannot use NSAIDs because of his cardiovascular history. He has been able to ambulate relatively well using a cane. Unfortunately, Mr. Jones fell down his stairs and re-injured his back. His pain is now more consistently in the 5/10 level. He would like to return to his baseline functional level.

He asks, "What can you offer me to help reduce the new pain and get me back on my feet again?"

Critical Analysis Questions

1. If some of the pain is related to a new compression fracture, what types of interventions would Mr. Jones be a candidate for? Does he meet the criteria for these techniques?

2. Would acupuncture be a good option to help Mr. Jones control his new pain?

3. Would SCS be a good choice to add to Mr. Jones' medication regimen? If so, why? If not, why?

4. If Mr. Jones had a pacemaker or defibrillator, would he be a good candidate for implanted techniques?

5. Which of these techniques would help Mr. Jones treat his new pain: epidural steroid injection, prolotherapy, epiduroscopy, IDET, SCS, or intrathecal pump implantation? Justify your choice.

8

PALLIATIVE CARE

Palliative care is often confused with end-of-life or hospice care. It is distinguished by its ability to coexist with curative options in the earlier stages of the illness, as the patient's disease begins to take an increasingly more significant toll on quality of life. The aim of palliative care is to maximize the quality of life for patients with progressive, chronic illness. Palliative care is not defined by the need for a "do not resuscitate" order or a 6-month time frame, and it is not dependent on the Medicare hospice benefit.

The research team who authored the 1995 Study to Understand Prognoses and Preferences for Outcomes and Risks of Treatments (SUPPORT) examined the status of Americans who were dying. The study revealed that 80% of Americans were dying in institutional settings—often in pain, isolated, on ventilatory support, and in intensive care units (Kuebler, Berry, & Heidrich, 2002). Health care providers and patients alike found the results to be quite unexpected and distressing. Most patients do not understand what will happen when they are admitted to the hospital and ask that "everything" be done. The result of the study was to bring focus to palliative care and end-of-life care and to highlight the positive effects that earlier intervention and symptom management can bring to the shifting of medical paradigms related to dying.

When patients opt for palliative care, it does not mean that they have given up hope and they view their health care provider as a failure for not curing them; rather, it means that the focus of care has shifted from curative options to the goals of symptom management and comfort. Table 8.1 compares curative care with palliative care.

TABLE 8.1 CURATIVE CARE VERSUS PALLIATIVE CARE

Curative Care	Palliative Care
Cure is the goal	Symptom control is the goal
Analytical and rationalistic	Subjective
Based on diagnosis	Based on symptoms
Scientific and biomedical	Humanistic and interpersonal
Aimed at disease process	Aimed at comfort
Views patients as parts	Views the patient as a whole
Based on "hard" science	Based on "soft" social sciences
Impersonal care	Individualized care
Death seen as a failure	Death accepted as normal

(Kuebler et al., 2002)

The definition of palliative care is conceptually broader than hospice care. Palliative care is "the active, total care of patients whose disease is not responsive to treatment (Kuebler et al., 2002; World Health Organization, 1990).

Palliative care focuses not only on the patient who is ill, but also on the family. It is designed to adapt to cultural needs and support the patient's ability to cope with chronic illness. It touches all aspects of the patient's life and the demands that chronic illness makes on social, psychosocial, financial, and spiritual domains.

Palliative care evolved from the oncology care setting into all areas of health care. Patients can include anyone with a progressive, chronic illness, such as

- Chronic pulmonary disease

- Chronic heart failure

- Neurological conditions, such as amyotrophic lateral sclerosis and Parkinson's disease

- HIV/AIDS

- Cardiac disease

- Chronic infections/sepsis/pneumonia

- Stroke

- Oncology diagnoses of all types

Many patients are referred to hospice care too late to benefit from the care and the support it can offer. One of the chief reasons why palliative care was developed, and why it has been successful, is that it is designed to intervene earlier in the disease process. Palliative care supports both the patient and family through the decision-making and natural physical decline of chronic illness. It offers support and symptom management.

THE PALLIATIVE CARE TEAM

The first hospital-based palliative care team was developed at McGill University in 1975 (Kuebler et al., 2002), and the concept has grown rapidly.

Not all palliative care teams look alike. Large institutions may organize a formal palliative care team, with attending physicians, residents, nurses, and ancillary staff who do daily rounding. Small hospitals may use a hospitalist model, with a hospitalist, nurse, and ancillary services such as social work, pharmacy, and chaplain's service. Whatever resources an institution can afford to apply to palliative care are beneficial to those patients who have reduced quality of life related to chronic illness. Members of a palliative care team can include, but are not limited to

- Health care providers (hospitalists, nurse practitioners, palliative care physicians)

- Nurses of all types (oncology, critical care, emergency department)

- Chaplains

- Social workers

- Outcomes management

- Nutritionists and dietitians

- Pharmacy staff

- Integrative medicine practitioners of all types (massage therapists, music therapists, healing touch practitioners)

Some fundamental elements of a palliative care team should be considered when developing the project. Most formal programs use a consult or unit-based model. The following elements are essential:

- Designate an "internal champion" for the palliative care team from within the health care facility. This person, who does not need to be a physician, is central to fostering buy-in from the staff.

- Provide continued follow-ups to increase patient satisfaction.

- Design interventions to help reduce patient length of stay.

- Continue to support the cultural shift in provider attitudes from the way it's always been done to the new palliative care mindset.

  (Oncology Watch, 2002)

Moving the care paradigm from a curative model to a supportive model is an unusual idea for some health care providers, who may feel as though they have failed the patient. Allowing palliative care practitioners to interact with members of the care team, patients, and family provides patients who are in the later stages of chronic illness a specialist who will focus on symptom management and quality-of-life issues.

The value of a palliative care team to a hospital, in addition to personal rewards for both caregivers and patients, can include

- Reduction in a patient's length of stay by moving patients to the correct level of care (e.g., from intensive care to a medical surgical or oncology unit with nurses trained in palliative care).

- Increased patient satisfaction because symptoms such as confusion, nausea, anxiety, fatigue, and swallowing and breathing difficulties are treated.

  (Oncology Watch, 2003)

Using palliative care reinforces the fact that patients who receive it reap benefits, even when the palliative care is combined with active therapy. Palliative care is designed as a value-added treatment option to help address symptom management at earlier stages, rather than waiting until acute care is needed (Whitecar, Maxwell, & Douglass, 2004).

Under Advisement

Palliative care practitioners should continue to include the primary-care attending physician and other members of the care team in care decisions. The palliative care involvement should be collaborative and value-added, and it should not displace the caregivers who have a long-standing relationship with the patient and his or her family.

Advance Directives

One of the most basic tenets of palliative care is to attempt to determine what patients at this stage of illness want for themselves now, and later as the disease progresses. An *advance directive* allows patients to indicate their desires regarding treatments and to designate a representative who will determine what actions will be taken if patients become incapacitated, unable to communicate, or unable to make decisions (Qaseem et al., 2008).

Advance directives can also be considered as living wills. The format is slightly different, but the intent is the same. In both instances patients indicate what types of treatment they would agree to if they were in an incapacitated state with a poor prognosis (e.g., nutrition, pain medication, ventilatory support). In the advance directive, the patient may also designate a health care decision maker for when the patient is no longer able to make decisions, often called the proxy for medical decisions. Some documents also may indicate who is to be in charge of financial decisions if the patient is unable to do so. The legal requirements for advance directives vary by state.

Five Wishes

Aging with Dignity, a Florida-based nonprofit organization, offers an advance directive known as Five Wishes (2009) available online at http://www.agingwithdignity.org/5wishes.html.

Patients record the following information:

1. The person they want to make health care decisions for them if they are unable to do so.
2. The kind of medical treatment they want or don't want.
3. How comfortable they want to be.
4. How they want people to treat them.
5. What they want their loved ones to know.

Gathering the salient information can be time-consuming and emotional. Some patients choose a formal approach to developing an advance directive, including seeking legal assistance, whereas other patients choose a more simplistic approach. Either way, an advance directive makes it easier for patients to approach the end of life on their own terms.

Symptom Management

If a patient with a chronic illness has declining function and quality of life, both the patient and family may experience grief and loss. Symptom management may be the key to providing the best possible quality of life for the patient, so that he or she can continue to interact with friends and family.

Many symptoms affect the quality of life for patients with chronic illness. Some symptoms are physical, such as respiratory distress or pain, and some symptoms are psychosocial, such as anxiety, denial, or spiritual distress. Palliative care practitioners must be prepared to deal not only with the physical aspects of the patient's needs, but also the deeper and more personal parts of the patient that may not be apparent.

Managing the adverse effects of a condition is easier when patients are able to report their symptoms. For patients who cannot report pain or anxiety, controlling symptoms is much more difficult. Other barriers also exist. Treatment for disease-related conditions, such as the inability to swallow, can limit the choice of treatment options. In each case, the choice to choose treatment or not is individualized to the particular patient's needs.

Physical Symptoms

Some patients who have chronic illness have a heavy physical symptom burden, while others do not. Many patients with cancer have pain management needs that palliative care can help meet. Other patients with respiratory disease such as chronic obstructive pulmonary disease

(COPD) or heart conditions such as chronic heart failure can have respiratory needs that should be addressed by aggressive treatment to avoid air hunger. The palliative care practitioner is skilled at dealing with the physical needs of the patient and helping the family to cope with pain, respiratory distress, or nutritional supplements.

Respiratory Distress

Some chronic illnesses, such as heart failure or lung cancer, can cause the patient to develop shortness of breath, or dyspnea. As the disease advances, the rates of dyspnea increase 50% to 75% (Kuebler et al., 2002). Patients describe dyspnea as shortness of breath, difficulty breathing or catching their breath, and a feeling of suffocation. Families have a difficult time seeing patients struggle to breathe, and a vicious circle of shortness of breath, anxiety, and feelings of helplessness can be shared by both patient and family members. As the problem worsens, the two groups can feed their anxiety about being unable to control the symptom to each other, increasing symptoms and the effect of the dyspnea.

Because dyspnea can adversely affect the patient's quality of life and ability to participate in daily activities, it is important to control it to the extent possible. The following treatments can help:

- **Supplemental oxygen** can be used to overcome the feelings of suffocation and inability to catch the breath (Qaseem et al., 2008). Most home oxygen companies cannot support the use of oxygen above 10 liters a minute.

- **Morphine** can be effective by blunting the perceptual response to the symptom (Kuebler et al., 2002). Recommendations for opioid-naïve patients start with up to 5 to 6mg of morphine every 4 hours, with increased doses for opioid-tolerant patients (Kuebler et al.). For older patients, reducing opioids by 25% to 50% (McLennon, 2005) with close observation is a good start.

- **Anxiolytics** such as benzodiazepine and phenothiazine are recommended for patients who become increasingly anxious as the shortness of breath develops. Examples of options include the following (Kuebler et al., 2002):

  - Lorazepam: 0.5mg every 4 to 6 hours, titrated to effect

  - Diazepam: 5 to 10mg immediately in a very anxious patient, and 2 to 5mg for older patients

  - Promethazine: 12.5mg every 4 to 6 hours and, as needed, titrated to effect

- **Steroids** should be used with care; dosing must be managed to avoid gastric irritation and bleeding, and fluid retention (Kuebler et al., 2002).

  - Prednisone: 30 to 60mg per day, with reduced doses for older patients

  - Dexamethasone: 6 to 8mg three to four times per day, with reduced doses for older patients

- **Bronchodilators** selected for the specific disease.

Pain

One of the primary goals for patients who elect palliative care is comfort. They may not have pain, but the prospect of experiencing pain is objectionable, and they want to indicate their wish for comfort even before pain is present. When pain is present in these patients, there are a wide variety of medications and interventional options that can provide relief.

Most palliative care patients who have pain are able to take oral medications. The regimen changes if the pain become constant or increases to the point that combination

For More Information

See Chapter 3 and Chapter 7 for additional information on medication and interventional treatments for pain.

medications such as oxycodone APAP or hydrocodone APAP titration reach toxic levels for acetaminophen. In that case, adding an extended-release medication such as extended-release oxycodone or extended-release morphine can help maintain adequate pain relief and lessen the need for shorter-acting pain medication.

Under Advisement

Opioid Dose Escalation

When a patient complains of decreased pain relief, the standard is to increase the dose by 25% to 100%, based on the patient's rating of the pain and overall condition. Doses may be increased from 50% to 100% in a 24-hour period for severe pain. Increases less than 25% are not usually effective. End point is reached when a decrease in pain is obtained or an intolerable side effect occurs. Older patients need careful dose titration and monitoring for side effects (Whitecar et al., 2004).

When a patient is placed on extended-release pain medication, it is important to provide adequate short-acting medication for breakthrough pain. Research indicates that older patients are able to sustain stable opioid doses over time, requiring fewer dose escalations and reporting lower pain scores after starting daily, long-acting opioid therapy (Buntin-Mushock, Phillip, Moriyama, & Palmer, 2005).

Patients who are on opioids for extended periods of time can become tolerant to the pain relief effect of the medications. In those cases, switching to another opioid may increase pain relief.

For More Information

Opioid rotation is the term given to the clinical practice of substituting one opioid for another in an attempt to achieve a better balance between pain relief and side effects (Quigley, 2006; D'Arcy, 2007).

Approximately 50% of patients who use opioid rotation show a clinical improvement in pain relief (Mercandante & Bruera, 2006). The usual method for conversion is to perform an equianalgesic conversion of the current opioid to the new opioid, and then decrease the new opioid dose by 25% to 50% (D'Arcy, 2007, Indelicato & Portnoy, 2002).

For example, MS Contin, 120mg total daily dose is equal to 80mg of the new medication OxyContin. The new medication can be decreased by 25% to 50% to a dose of 40 to 60mg to start. The patient is offered breakthrough medication to preserve adequate pain relief.

Bone Pain/Neuropathic Pain

Bone Pain

Bone pain that is the result of bone metastases can be treated with an infusion of a bisphosphonate such as pamidronate. A single infusion of pamidronate can inhibit osteoclast activity for an extended period of time—weeks or months. Radiopharmaceuticals such as strontium 89 can also help decrease bone pain, as it is absorbed into areas of high bone turnover and does not affect marrow suppression (Kuebler et al., 2002).

Neuropathic Pain

Chemotherapy with platin and vinca alkaloid drugs can produce a neuropathic pain that affects the hands and feet in a stocking glove distribution. To treat this type of pain, a coanalgesic that is effective for neuropathic pain is needed. Opioids alone will not fully control this type of pain. Using a gabapentin, pregabalin, or antidepressant medication in conjunction with opioid or non-opioid medications can provide extra pain relief and decrease the painful neuropathic sensations.

For patients who are closer to end of life and have elected a comfort care or terminal care status, additional options to control pain can be used, including continuous opioid drips and adjunct medication such as anti-anxiety drugs. (See Figure 8.1)

Nutritional Needs

Patients with a chronic illness need extra calories to cope with the high energy requirements. For example, pulmonary patients need a higher caloric intake to compensate for the additional calories required to breathe effectively. Some cancer patients can develop *cachexia* (physical wasting) or *anorexia* (loss of appetite; Kuebler et al., 2002). Because most patients with chronic illness require extra nutrition, the interventions for this condition focus on providing extra calories.

To help patients who have a nutritional deficit, consider some of the following recommendations:

- Refer to a dietitian for suggestions about meals and supplements.

- Offer patients a choice of their favorite foods.

- Offer small meals frequently.

- Use high protein supplements, as needed.

The following medications can be used to stimulate the appetite, although their success rates vary from patient to patient:

- Megestrol acetate (Megace)

- Corticosteroids

- Metoclopramide (Reglan)

- Cannabinoids

As with all other medications, when used in older patients, drug-drug interactions and careful dosing should be observed.

The decision to use an *enteral feeding device* is always controversial. Before using this intervention, a careful discussion of risks and benefits should take place with the patient and family. Although a *gastrostomy tube* can provide the needed nutrition, it can also result in aspiration pneumonia and diarrhea. Enteral feedings are not recommended for patients who have developed cachexia (Kuebler et al., 2002). However, enteral feedings can provide the needed nutrition to patients who have a neurological condition that impairs swallowing, such as patients who have had a stroke, as well as to patients who have an appetite but have a physical barrier to eating, such as patients with head and neck cancers.

SUBURBAN HOSPITAL
Healthcare System

COMFORT CARE PHYSICIAN ORDERS

ALLERGIES ➤

I HEREBY AUTHORIZE THE PHARMACY TO DISPENSE A GENERIC EQUIVALENT
UNLESS THE PARTICULAR DRUG IS CIRCLED.

PATIENT PLATE

Please check all boxes on orders that are wanted. If the box is not checked the order will not be activated.

Advance Directives
- ☐ Advance directives on chart
- ☐ If no advance directives:

Surrogate identified _____

   Relationship _____

   Telephone number _____

Vital Signs/Activity

Vital signs (BP, heart rate, respirations): ☐ every ___ hours
        ☐ every ___ hours only while awake

Temperature: ☐ every ___ hours   ☐ every ___ hours only while awake
        ☐ discontinue routine temperatures

Activity: ☐ as tolerated   ☐ bedrest   ☐ out of bed

Respiratory Therapy
- ☐ Oxygen
  - _____ Liters/minute via nasal cannula ☐ prn dyspnea
  - _____ F₁O₂ high humidity mask/collar/T-piece
  - _____ 100% non-rebreather mask ☐ prn dyspnea
  - _____ F₁O₂ venturi mask ☐ prn dyspnea
- ☐ Nasotracheal suctioning as needed

Diet/Hydration
- ☐ Diet _____

- ☐ Intravenous fluids _____ at ___ ml/hr
- ☐ Saline lock IV   ☐ Discontinue IV
- ☐ Fluids via nasogastric tube _____ (see tube feeding order form.)
- ☐ Nasogastric tube to: ☐ low continuous suction ☐ low intermittent suction
          ☐ gravity drainage
- ☐ Discontinue nasogastric tube/orogastric tube/feeding tube

Consults
- ☐ Social services for hospice and/or discharge planning
- ☐ Pain Nurse Specialist
- ☐ Palliative care* Requires MD order
- ☐ Pastoral care
- ☐ Wound Ostomy Care Nurse
- ☐ Nutrition

Hygiene/Other Comfort Measures
- ☐ Turn and position for comfort and skin care every 2 hours and prn
- ☐ Activate "pressure relief" mode on bed
- ☐ Mouth care every four hours
- ☐ Monitor for fecal impaction every day and evacuate as necessary
- ☐ Foley catheter
- ☐ Discontinue DVT prophylaxis
- ☐ Discontinue all labs and blood glucose finger sticks
- ☐ Discontinue weights
- ☐ Discontinue pulse oximetry
- ☐ Private room
- ☐ Unlimited family visitation

Other _____

Medications
- ☐ Discontinue the following medications: _____

- ☐ Discontinue all PO meds (when the patient's ability to swallow is compromised).

Fever
- ☐ Tylenol (acetaminophen) 650 mg ☐ PO ☐ PR every ___ hrs prn temperature ≥ 101°
- ☐ Motrin (ibuprofen) ☐ 400mg ☐ every ___ hr ☐ prn **OR** ☐ 600mg PO every ___ hr ☐ prn
- ☐ Other _____

Anxiety/Agitation/Restlessness
- ☐ Ativan (lorazepam) ☐ 0.5mg ☐ 1mg ☐ 2mg   ☐ PO ☐ IV every ___ hrs ☐ prn
- ☐ Ativan (lorazepam) (1mg/ml) at ___ ml/hr IV. Increase by ___ ml every ___ minutes prn agitation.

Pain
- ☐ Percocet (oxycodone 5mg/acetaminophen 325 mg) ☐ 1 tab ☐ 2 tabs PO every ___ hrs ☐ prn
- ☐ OxyContin (oxycodone extended release) ___ mg PO every ___ hrs
- ☐ OxyIR (oxycodone immediate release) ___ mg PO every ___ prn breakthrough pain

- ☐ MSIR (morphine immediate release) ___ mg PO every ___ hrs prn breakthrough pain
- ☐ MS Contin (morphine extended release) ___ mg PO every ___ hrs
- ☐ Morphine solution ☐ 5mg ☐ 10mg ☐ PO ☐SL ___ every ___ hr(s) prn pain or dyspnea
- ☐ Morphine sulfate ___ mg IV every ___ hr(s) prn pain or dyspnea
- ☐ Morphine (1mg/ml) continuous infusion for pain or for dyspnea: See opioid titration orders.

- ☐ Dilaudid (hydromorphone) ___ mg PO every ___ hrs ☐ prn
- ☐ Dilaudid (hydromorphone) (1mg/ml) continuous infusion for pain: See opioid titration orders.

- ☐ Duragesic (fentanyl) transdermal patch ___ micrograms/hr to be changed every 72 hours
- ☐ Sublimaze (fentanyl) (5mcg/ml) continuous infusion for pain: See opioid titration orders.

Adjuvant Pain Medications
- ☐ Decadron (dexamethasone) ___ mg   ☐ PO ☐ IV   every ___ hrs ☐ prn
- ☐ Toradol (ketorolac) ☐ 15mg ☐ 30mg IV every ___ hrs ☐prn (maximum number of doses = ___)

Nausea /Vomiting
- ☐ Zofran (ondansetron hydrochloride) ☐ 4mg ☐ 8mg IV   every ___ hrs   ☐ prn
- ☐ Reglan (metoclopramide) 10mg ☐ PO ☐ IV   every ___ hrs   ☐ prn
- ☐ Phenergan (promethazine hydrochloride) ☐ 12.5mg ☐ 25mg ☐ PR ☐ IV every ___ hrs ☐ prn

General Comfort
- ☐ Benadryl (diphenhydramine) ☐ 25mg ☐ 50mg ☐ PO ☐ IV   every ___ hrs prn itching
- ☐ Dulcolax (bisacodyl) 1 suppository PR QD prn
- ☐ Senokot (senna) 2 tablets PO BID prn
- ☐ Fleets enema prn

Other medications (specify drug, dose, route) _____

SIGNATURE   TITLE   DATE   TIME   PRINTED   SIGNATURE   TITLE   DATE   TIME   PRINTED

MEDICAL RECORDS

SUBURBAN HOSPITAL
Healthcare System
8600 Old Georgetown Road
Bethesda, Maryland 20814
COMFORT CARE PHYSICIAN'S ORDERS
FORM 1-1150 (10/03)

FIGURE 8.1   COMFORT CARE PHYSICIAN ORDERS

SUBURBAN HOSPITAL
Healthcare System

COMFORT CARE PHYSICIAN ORDERS
Intravenous Opioid Titration Orders

ALLERGIES ➤	

PATIENT PLATE

OPIOID:

☐ Morphine (1mg/ml)
☐ Dilaudid (hydromorphone) (1mg/ml)
☐ Sublimaze (fentanyl) (5mcg/ml)

Opioid Naïve Patients:

☐ Loading bolus _____ ml
  Suggested: Morphine 2 milligrams, Dilaudid 0.5 milligrams, Fentanyl 25 micrograms
☐ Continuous infusion at _____ ml/hr
  Assess pain every   ☐ 15 minutes   ☐ 30 minutes   until pain score is < 4 (or at a level tolerable to the patient).
    If pain score is < 4, no change.
    If pain score is 4 to 5, increase infusion rate by _____ mg (suggested 25% increase)*
    If pain score is 6 to 7, increase infusion rate by _____ mg (suggested 50% increase)*
    If pain score is > 7, increase infusion rate by _____ mg (suggested 100% increase)*
    Bolus dose _____ mg for breakthrough pain (suggested 25% of continuous infusion rate)*
    *Dosage to be confirmed by 2 nurses.
  Once pain is controlled (pain score < 4 and at a level tolerable to the patient), continue pain assessments every 4 hours
  and prn.

Opioid Tolerant Patients:

  Convert p.o. opioid dose to IV equivalent _____ **
☐ Loading bolus _____ ml
☐ Continuous infusion at _____ ml/hr
  Assess pain every   ☐ 30 minutes   ☐ 60 minutes   until pain score is < 4 (or at a level tolerable to the patient).
    If pain score is < 4, no change.
    If pain score is 4 to 5, increase infusion rate by _____ mg (suggested 25% increase)**
    If pain score is 6 to 7, increase infusion rate by _____ mg (suggested 50% increase)**
    If pain score is > 7, increase infusion rate by _____ mg (suggested 100% increase)**
    Bolus dose _____ mg for breakthrough pain (suggested 25% of continuous infusion rate)**
    **Dosage to be confirmed by 2 nurses and a pharmacist.
  Once pain is controlled (pain score < 4 and at a level tolerable to the patient), continue pain assessments every 4 hours
  and prn.

SIGNATURE	TITLE	DATE	TIME	PRINTED	SIGNATURE	TITLE	DATE	TIME	PRINTED

FIGURE 8.1 (CONTINUED)

PSYCHOSOCIAL SYMPTOMS

Some patients have intense psychosocial needs that surpass any physical symptoms they may have. Unresolved family relationships, grief at leaving loved ones, spiritual distress, or depression as the result of feeling helpless or hopeless can be more difficult to treat than pain. This group of symptoms may need a combined effort by chaplains, counselors, psychologists, and social workers trained in dealing with coping and grief. By using an interdisciplinary approach to symptom management, the patients and family may be able to resolve current issues and come together and experience a higher level of quality of life for both the patient and family members.

Depression

Depression is a common symptom among patients who struggle daily with the disability and chronicity of a long-term illness. The depression is not often classed as clinical, but more often considered to be reactive or situational, which tends to be self-limiting once the patient receives support, education, and medication, if needed.

Standard assessment tools for depression include the following:

- **Beck Depression Inventory (BDI):** A reliable and valid tool that can identify subtypes of depression and differentiate anxiety from depression (Beck, Steer, & Carbin, 1988).

- **Geriatric Depression Scale (GDS):** A simple 15-item scale used as a screening tool for depression in older adults (Brown, Woods, & Storandt, 2007).

> **Clinical Tip**
>
> For patients in palliative care, a suicide assessment can help determine if symptoms have reached a point to where the patient feels he or she has lost control, and suicide might be considered as an option to end suffering.

- **Brief Symptom Inventory (BSI):** A tool with nine subscales (e.g., depression, anxiety, hostility) that can be used to study changes in the subscale over time (Long, Harring, Brekke, Test, & Greenberg, 2007).

Treating depression requires a multimodal plan of intervention that can include psychotherapy, counseling, coping strategies, medications, integrative medicine techniques, and spiritual support (Qaseem et al., 2008).

The following antidepressant medications can be used to help lessen depression:

- **Selective serotonin reuptake inhibitors (SSRIs):** citalopram, fluoxetine, paroxetine, escitalopram oxalate, fluvoamine, and sertraline

- **Serotonin-norepinephrine reuptake inhibitors (SNRIs):** venlafaxine, duloxetine, and desvenlafaxine

- **Norepinephrine-dopamine reuptake inhibitor (NDRI):** bupropion HCl
  (Kuebler et al., 2002)

Tricyclic antidepressants are not recommended for the elderly due to their adverse side effects (Kuebler et al., 2002).

As with opioid medications, the older patient needs careful assessment and evaluation when starting antidepressant medications. Drug-drug interactions should be reviewed, and doses should be adjusted until the patient's toleration is ascertained.

Anxiety

Anxiety is defined as feelings of vague apprehension or uneasiness, often accompanied by feelings of uncertainty and helplessness (Kuebler et al., 2002). Anxiety is not a static condition; it can range from mild to severely disabling or panic attacks. For mild anxiety, an anxiolytic, taken as needed, may be sufficient to control the symptom. For more severe cases of anxiety, psychiatric intervention with medication management may be needed. Patients who might be at higher risk of experiencing anxiety include patients with cancer, pulmonary, or neurologic diseases.

Medications that can be used to treat and reduce anxiety include the following:

- **Benzodiazepines:** lorazepam, alprazolam, diazepam

- **Neuroleptics:** haloperidol

- **Antihistamines:** hydroxyzine, diphenhydramine
  (Kuebler et al., 2002)

THE GOOD DEATH

Most patients who are diagnosed with a chronic illness fear the diagnosis, but do not fully understand the full spectrum of the impact it will have on them. Once they understand the full effect of the disease on their lives, patients may adjust, become angry, avoid the idea with denial, or compromise. Regardless of the coping style, managing the symptoms to help maintain functionality and quality of life is central to end-of-life care.

Eventually, the patient will start considering the "what-ifs." What if I could get better? What if I don't get better? For most patients with a chronic illness, the illness trajectory will trend downward with increasing functional impairment that is totally dependent on treatment options, the type of disease, the health status of the patients before they became ill, and their willingness to participate in health-promoting, therapeutic options such as physical therapy. For older patients, there may be more acceptance of their condition, but also more anxiety as it threatens their ability to live and function independently.

Grieving over the loss of mobility and independence is common. Loss of abilities and role status in families can be very upsetting to older patients. Eventually, they will begin to adjust to the concept of managing the symptoms of their disease rather than expecting a cure. For some patients this process may take years—for others, a matter of months. No matter how long it takes, the patient will eventually look for the "good death"—one that is pain-free and where all the symptoms can be managed.

The Nurse's Role

Nurses have an integral role in helping both patients and their families. They must recognize that patients and families have expended physical and emotional energy while coping with a chronic illness for an extended period of time. Participating in the care of a patient with the family who has cared for him or her for many years requires a special type of collaboration that reaches into every aspect of the patient's life. It is a close and emotional type of care that can be very rewarding and yet emotionally taxing.

Active listening and thoughtful communication are two essential elements for nurses who care for patients receiving palliative or end-of-life care. Families often tell nurses what the patient likes and does not like, what works for pain, or what works for anxiety. They share tidbits of information about the patient's life and interests. Listening attentively and responding thoughtfully to these pieces of information are important for preserving the patient's "personhood," the very essence of who they are.

Thoughtful communication can encompass many different styles of interaction with the patient and family; it includes not only verbal communication, but also physical interaction—the way the patient is touched or moved. Families take comfort in knowing that their family member is receiving care from professionals who are dedicated to making him or her feel comfortable and valued.

Families often ask nurses about diagnoses, prognosis, test results, and treatment options. Some nurses are reluctant to discuss these topics with the patient or family. However, families report that these discussions give them comfort and information that is very important to them. Providing this communication is a gift that nurses can give to patients and families when there is little to offer in the way of therapy.

To improve their communication skills, nurses can participate in role-playing exercises. One nurse can play the patient or family member, while another nurse plays the nurse caring for the patient. Watching how other nurses respond to patient and family questions can help prepare nurses for the actual conversations that will take place with their patients.

SUMMARY

Palliative care is a way to manage symptoms that accompany a chronic illness. Preparing for end of life with an advance directive and intervening early with palliative care options can help to preserve quality of life. Palliative care requires specialized nursing interventions. Providing symptom management, emotional care, spiritual care, and a variety of treatment options along with good communication skills, will help patients find the "good death" they seek.

CASE STUDY

Sally Sims is a 78-year-old patient who has chronic heart failure. Her ejection fraction has been slowly decreasing and is at 20%. She has had repeated hospitalizations for shortness of breath and fluid retention. Each time she has been given a diuretic and sent home, only to return for shortness of breath. Her husband is anxious about his wife's worsening condition. Both Sally and her husband want her to remain at home, but it is becoming too difficult to manage. They ask if there are any services that could help them maintain the quality of life Sally would like and to remain in their home.

In addition to heart failure, Sally has osteoarthritis, diabetes, and hypertension. She has made out an advance directive that appoints her husband as her power of attorney for health care decisions, and she has indicated that she wishes to receive a full code, nutritional supplementation, if needed, and enough pain medication to keep her comfortable, even though it could potentially shorten her life. The attending physician asks the palliative care specialist to see Sally to determine if symptom management can help Sally remain at home with her husband as her illness progresses.

Since Sally can be a full partner in discharge planning, a care team and family meeting is held. The interventions that the health care team put in place for Sally before her discharge include

- Nutrition consult to assess the type of diet and nutritional supplements Sally has been using. Education is provided to both Sally and her husband about the need for a low-sodium, diabetic diet.

- Home oxygen is ordered to help Sally breathe better at night.

- Adequate pain medication is used to help Sally with osteoarthritis pain. Anxiolytics are provided for anxiety when she gets short of breath.

- Sally agrees to try some relaxation and meditation techniques to help her relax when her breathing gets difficult.

- Although Sally and her husband can no longer attend church, a remote hook-up is arranged so Sally and her husband can hear Sunday services via their phone.

- A home visiting nursing service is ordered, with regular follow-up visits that include weighing Sally, taking her blood pressure, and monitoring her glucose.

- A volunteer service is contacted to provide Sally's husband with regular respite care for Sally, so he can attend some monthly group meetings with his friends in local organizations that he has been missing.

Although Sally's disease progresses to the point that she becomes oxygen-dependent, she is able to stay at home and enjoy her remaining days with her husband.

Critical Analysis Questions

1. Should Sally have had palliative care earlier in her illness? What benefits would there have been to an earlier intervention with palliative care?

2. What other options would have been helpful for treating Sally's chronic illness?

3. Develop a comprehensive medication and care plan for Sally, using the medications and techniques discussed in the chapter.

4. What are some essential elements of an advance directive?

5. What types of interventions and interactions would the nurse caring for Sally need to provide for effective care?

REFERENCES

CHAPTER 1

American Geriatrics Society (AGS). (2002). The management of persistent pain in older persons. *Journal of the American Geriatrics Society*, *50*, S205-S224.

American Health Care Association (AHCA). (n.d.). *Nursing home statistics*. Retrieved 17 September 2009 from http://www.efmoody.com/longterm/nursingstatistics.html

American Pain Society (APS). (2008). *Principles of analgesic use in the treatment of acute pain and cancer pain*. Glenview, IL: Author.

Bruckenthal, P., & D'Arcy, Y. (2007). Assessment and management of pain in older adults: A review of the basics. *Topics in Advanced Practice Nursing ejournal 2007*(1). Retrieved 17 September 2009 from http://www.medscape.com/viewarticle/556382

D'Arcy, Y. (2007). *Pain management: Evidence-based tools and techniques for nursing professionals*. Marblehead, MA: HcPro.

D'Arcy, Y. (2009a). Be in the know about pain management. *The Nurse Practitioner Journal*, *34*(4), 43-47.

D'Arcy, Y. (2009b). Overturning barriers to pain relief in older adults. *Nursing 2009*, *39*(10), 32-39.

Hadjistavropoulos, T., Herr, K., Turk, D. C., Fine, P. G., Dworkin, R. H., & Helme, R., et al. (2007). An interdisciplinary expert consensus statement on assessment of pain in older persons. *Clinical Journal of Pain*, *23*(1), S1-S43.

McLennon, S. M. (2005). *Persistent pain management*. University of Iowa Gerontological Nursing Interventions Research Center. Retrieved 3 August 2009 from http://www.guideline.gov

Smeltzer, S., Bare, B., Hinkle, J., & Cheever, K. (2008). *Textbook of medical-surgical nursing*. Philadelphia: Lippincott Williams & Wilkins.

St. Marie, B. (Ed.) (2002). *Core curriculum for pain management nursing*. Philadelphia: W. B. Saunders.

CHAPTER 2

American Geriatrics Society (AGS). (2002). The management of persistent pain in older persons. *Journal of the American Geriatrics Society, 50*, S205-S224.

American Pain Society (APS). (2009). *Principles of analgesic use in the treatment of acute and cancer pain* (6th ed.). Glenview, IL: American Pain Society.

American Society for Pain Management Nursing (ASPMN). (2009). *Core curriculum for pain management nursing*. Philadelphia: Saunders.

Bruckenthal, P., & D'Arcy, Y. (2007). Pain in the older adult. *Topics in Advanced Practice ejournal*. Retrieved 1 April 2008 from http://www.medscape.com

Chok, B. (1998). An overview of the visual analogue scale and the McGill pain questionnaire. *Physiotherapy Singapore, 1*(3), 88-93.

Dahl, J., & Kehlet, H. (2006). Postoperative pain and its management. In McMahon, S.B., & Koltzenburg, M. (Eds.), *Wall and Melzack's textbook of pain* (5th ed.). Philadelphia: Churchill Livingstone.

D'Arcy, Y. (2003). Pain assessment. In P. Iyer (Ed.), *Medical-legal aspects of pain and suffering*. Tucson, AZ: Lawyers and Judges Publishing Company.

D'Arcy, Y. (2007a). What's the diagnosis? *American Nurse Today, 1*(4).

D'Arcy, Y. (2007b). *Pain management: Evidence-based tools and techniques for nursing professionals*. Marblehead, MA: HcPro.

Daut, R. L., Cleeland, C. S., & Flannery, R. (1983). Development of the Wisconsin brief pain questionnaire to assess pain in cancer or other diseases. *Pain, 17*, 197-210.

Feldt, K. S. (2000). The checklist of non-verbal pain indicators (CNPI). *Pain Management Nursing, 1*(1), 13-21.

Feldt, K. S., Ryden, M. B., & Miles, S. (1998). Treatment of pain in cognitively impaired compared with cognitively intact older patients with hip fractures. *Journal of the American Geriatrics Society, 46*, 1079-1085.

Ger, L., Ho, S., Sun, W., Wang, M., & Cleeland, C. (1999). Validation of the brief pain inventory in a Taiwanese population. *Journal of Pain and Symptom Management, 18*(5), 316-22.

Gordon, D., Pellino, T., Miaskowski, C., McNeill, J. A., Paice, J., & Laferriere, D., et al. (2002). A 10-year review of quality improvement monitoring in pain management: Recommendations for standardized outcome measures. *Pain Management Nursing, 3*(4), 116-130.

Gracely, R. H. (1992). Evaluation of multi-dimensional pain scales. *Pain, 48*(3), 297-300.

Graham, C., Bond, S., Gerkovich, M., & Cook, M. (1980). Use of the McGill pain questionnaire in the assessment of cancer pain: Replicability and consistency. *Pain, 8*, 377-387.

Hadjistavropoulos, T., Herr, K., Turk, D., Fine, P., Dworkin, R., & Helme, et al. (2007). An interdisciplinary expert consensus statement on assessment of pain in older persons. *Clinical Journal of Pain, 23*(1), S1-S43.

Herr, K. A., & Mobily, P. (1993). Comparison of selected pain assessment tools for use with the elderly. *Applied Nursing Research 6*(1), 39-46.

Herr, K., Bjoro, K., & Decker, S. (2006). Tools for assessment of pain in nonverbal older adults with dementia: A state-of-the-science review. *Journal of Pain and Symptom Management, 31*(2), 170-192.

Jensen, M. P. (2003). The validity and reliability of pain measures in adults with cancer. *The Journal of Pain 4*(1), 2-21.

Joint Commission on Accreditation of Healthcare Organizations. (JCAHO; 2000). *Pain assessment and management: An organizational approach*. Oakbrook Terrace, IL: JCAHO.

Joint Commission on Accreditation of Healthcare Organizations (JCAHO; 2005, October). Focus on five: Preventing patient controlled analgesia overdose. *Joint Commission Perspectives on Patient Safety.*

Klepstad, P., Loge, J. H., Borchgrevink, P. C., Mendoza, T. R., Cleeland, C., & Kaasa, S. (2002). The Norwegian brief pain inventory questionnaire: Translation and validation in cancer pain patients. *Journal of Pain and Symptom Management, 24*(5), 517-525.

Lane, P., Kuntupis, M., MacDonald, S., McCarthy, P., Panke, J. A., Warden, V., et al. (2003). A pain assessment tool for people with advanced Alzheimer's and other progressive dementias. *Home Healthcare Nurse, 21*(1), 32-37.

McDonald, D. D., & Weiskopf. C. S. A. (2001). Adult patients' postoperative pain descriptions and responses to the short form McGill pain questionnaire. *Clinical Nursing Research, 10*(4), 442-452.

McIntyre, D. L., Hopkins, P. M., & Harris, S. R. (1995). Evaluation of pain and functional activity in patellofemoral pain syndrome: Reliability and validity of two assessment tools. *Physiotherapy of Canada, 47*(3), 164-170.

Melzack, R. (1975). The McGill pain questionnaire: Major properties and scoring methods. *Pain, 1*, 277–299.

Melzack, R. (1987). The short form McGill pain questionnaire, *Pain, 30*, 191-197.

Mystakidou, K., Parpa E., Tsilika, E., Kalaidopoulou, O., Georgaki, S., Galanos, A., et al. (2002). Greek McGill pain questionnaire: Validation and utility in cancer patients. *Journal of Pain and Symptom Management, 24*(4), 370-387.

Radbruch, L., Liock, G., Kiencke, P., Lindena, G., Sabatowski, R., Grond, S., et al. (1999). Validation of the German version of the brief pain inventory. *Journal of Pain and Symptom Management, 18* (3), 180-187.

Raiche, K. A., Osborne, T. L., Jensen, M. P., & Cardenas D. (2006). The reliability and validity of pain interference measures in persons with spinal cord injury. Journal of Pain, 7(3), 179-186.

Staats, P. S., Argoff, C., Brewer, R., D'Arcy, Y., Gallagher, R., McCarberg, W., et al. (2004). Neuropathic pain: Incorporating new consensus guidelines into the reality of clinical practice. *Advanced Studies in Medicine, 4*(7B), S542-582.

Tan, G., Jensen, M. P., Thornby, J. I., & Shanti, B. F. (2004). Validation of the brief pain inventory for chronic non-malignant pain. *Journal of Pain and Symptom Management, 5*(2), 133-137.

Tittle, M. B., McMillan, S.C., & Hagan, S. (2003). Validating the brief pain inventory for use with surgical patients with cancer. *Oncology Nursing Forum, 30*(2), 325-330.

Weiner, D., Herr, K., & Rudy, T. E. (Eds.). (2002). *Persistent pain in older adults: An interdisciplinary guide for treatment*. New York: Springer.

Williams V. S. L., Smith, M. Y., & Fehnel, S. E. (2006). The validity and utility of the BPI interference measures for evaluating the impact of osteoarthritis pain. *Journal of Pain and Symptom Management, 31*(1), 48–57.

CHAPTER 3

Adams, M., & Abdieh, H. (2004). Pharmokinetics and dose proportionality of oxymorphone extended release and its metabolites: Results of a randomized crossover study. *Pharmacotherapy, 24*(4), 468-476.

Adams, M., Pienaszek, H., Gammatoni, A., & Abdieh, H. (2005). Oxymorphone extended release does not affect CVP2C9 or CYP3A4 metabolite pathways. *Journal of Clinical Pharmacology, 45*, 337-345.

American Geriatrics Society (AGS). (2002). The management of persistent pain in older persons. *Journal of the American Geriatrics Society, 50*, S205-S224.

American Geriatrics Society (AGS). (2009). Pharmacological management of persistent pain in older persons. *Journal of the American Geriatrics Society, 57*, 1331-1346.

Antman, E. M., Bennett, J. S., Daugherty, A., Furberg, C., Roberts, H., & Taubert, K. A. (2007). Use of nonsteroidal anti-inflammatory drugs. An update for clinicians. A scientific statement from the American Heart Association. *Circulation, 115*.

American Pain Society (APS). (2009). *Principles of analgesic use in the treatment of acute pain and cancer pain*. Glenview, IL: Author.

American Academy of Pain Medicine, American Pain Society, and American Society of Addiction Medicine. (2001). *Advocacy. Definitions related to the use of opioids for the treatment of pain*. Retrieved 12 November 2009 from http://www.ampainsoc.org/advocacy/opioids2.htm

Bennett, J. S., Daugherty, A., Herrington, D., Greenland, P., Roberts, H., & Taubert, K. A. (2005). The use of nonsteroidal anti-inflammatory drugs (NSAIDs): A science advisory from the American Heart Association. *Circulation, 111*, 1713-1716.

Berry, P., Covington, E., Dahl, J., Katz, J., & Miaskowski, C. (2006). *Pain: Current understanding of assessment, management, and treatments*. Reston, VA: National Pharmaceutical Council, Inc.

Bruckenthal, P., & D'Arcy, Y. (2007). Assessment and management of pain in older adults: A review of the basics. *Topics in Advanced Practice Nursing ejournal, 7*(1). Retrieved 13 July 2009 from http://www.medscape.com/viewarticle/556382

Capone, M. L., Sciulli, M. G., Tacconelli, S., Grana, M, Ricciotti, E., Renda, G., et al. (2005). Pharmacodynamic interaction of naproxen with low-dose aspirin in healthy subjects. *Journal of the College of Cardiology, 45*, 1295-1301.

Catella-Lawson, F., Reilly, M. P., Kapoor S. C., Cucchiara, A. J., DeMarco, S., Tournier, B. et al. (2001). Cyclooxygenase inhibitors and the antiplatelet effects of aspirin. *New England Journal of Medicine, 345*, 1809-1817.

Chou, R., Fanciullo, G., Fine, P., Adler, J., Ballantyne, J., Davies, P., et al. (2009). Opioid treatment guidelines: Clinical guidelines for the use of chronic opioid therapy in chronic noncancer pain. *The Journal of Pain, 10*(2), 113-130.

Dahl, J., & Kehlet, H. (2006). Postoperative pain and its managememnt. In S. B. McMahom, & M. Koltzenburg (Eds.), *Wall and Melzack's Textbook of Pain* (5th ed.). Philadelphia: Churchill Livingstone.

Dalton, J. A., & Youngblood, R. (2001). Clinical application of the World Health Organization analgesic ladder. *Journal of Intravenous Nursing, 23*(2), 118-124.

D'Arcy, Y. (2007). Pain management: Evidence-based tools and techniques for nursing professionals. Marblehead, MA: HcPro.

D'Arcy, Y. (2008). Pain in the older adult. *The Nurse Practitioner, 33*(3), 19-24.

Fine, P., & Portnoy, R. (2007). *A clinical guide to opioid analgesia.* New York: Vendome Group.

Horgas, A. (2003). Pain management in elderly adults. *Journal of Infusion Nursing, 26*(3), 161-165.

Huffman, J., & Kunik, M. (2000). Assessment and understanding of pain in patients with dementia. *The Gerontologist, 40*(5), 574-581.

Karani, R., & Meier, D. (2004). Systematic pharmacologic postoperative pain management in the geriatric orthopedic patients. *Clinical Orthopedics & Related Research, 425,* 26-34.

Løvlie, R., Daly, A. K., Matre, G. E., Molven, A., & Steen, V. M. (2001). Polymorphisms in CYP2D6 duplication-negative individuals with the ultrarapid metabolizer phenotype: A role for the CYP2D6*35 allele in ultrarapid metabolism? *Pharmacogenetics, 11*(1), 45-55.

McLennon, S. M. (2005). Persistent pain management. National Guidelines Clearinghouse. Retrieved 1 April 2008 from http://www.guideline.gov

Perez-Gutthann, S., Rodiriguez, L. A., & Raifoed, D. S. (1997). Individual nonsteroidal anti-inflammatory drugs and other risk factors for upper gastrointestinal bleeding and perforation. *Epidemiology, 8,* 18-24.

Potter, J. (2004). The older orthopedic patient: General considerations. *Clinical Orthopedics & Related Research, 425,* 4-49.

Sturkenboom, M. C., Burke, T. A., Tangelder, M. J. D., Dieleman, J., Walton, S., & Goldstein, J. (2003). Adherence to proton pump inhibitors or H2-receptor antagonists during the use of non-steroidal anti-inflammatory drugs. *Alimentary Pharmacology and Therapeutics, 18,* 1137-1147.

Wallace, M. S., & Staats, P. (2005). *Pain medicine and management.* New York: McGraw-Hill.

Warltier, D., Chassard, D., & Bruguerolle, B. (2004). Chronobiology and anesthesia. *Anesthesiology, 100*(2), 413-427.

Zurakowski, T. (2009). The practicalities and pitfalls of polypharmacy. *The Nurse Practitioner, 34*(4), 36-41.

CHAPTER 4

American Geriatrics Society (AGS). (2002). The management of persistent pain in older persons-The American Geriatrics Society panel on persistent pain in older persons. *Journal of the American Geriatrics Society, 50*(6), 205-224.

American Pain Society (APS). (2002). *Guideline for the management of pain in osteoarthritis, rheumatoid arthritis, and juvenile chronic arthritis.* Glenview, IL: American Pain Society.

American Pain Society (APS). (2005). *Guideline for the management of fibromyalgia pain syndrome in adults and children.* Glenview, IL: American Pain Society.

American Pain Society (APS). (2006). *Pain control in the primary care setting.* Glenview, IL: American Pain Society.

American Society of Pain Management Nurses (ASPMN). (2002). *Core curriculum for pain management Nursing.* Philadelphia: WB Saunders.

Berry, P., Covington, E., Dahl, J., Katz, J., & Miaskowski, C. (2006). *Pain: Current understanding of assessment, management, and treatments.* Reston, VA: National Pharmaceutical Council, Inc.

Bruckenthal, P., & D'Arcy, Y. (2007). A complementary approach to pain management. *Topics in Advanced Practice Nursing eJournal, 7*(1). Retrieved 30 May 2007 from http://www.medscape.com/viewarticle/556408

Chou, R., & Huffman, L. (2007). Nonpharmacologic therapies for acute and chronic low back pain : A review of the evidence for an American Pain Society/American College of physicians clinical practice guideline. *Annals of Internal Medicine, 147*(7), 492-504.

The Cochrane Collaboration. (n.d.) *About the Cochrane collaboration.* Retrieved 15 August 2009 from http://www.cochrane.org/docs/descrip.htm

Cole, B. H., & Brunk, Q. (1999). Holistic interventions for acute pain episodes: An integrative review. *Journal of Holistic Nursing, 17*(4), 384–96.

D'Arcy, Y. (2007). Pain management: *Evidence-based tools and techniques for nursing professionals.* Marblehead, MA: HcPro, Inc.

Dillard, J., & Knapp, S. (2005). Complementary and alternative pain therapy in the emergency department. *Emergency Medical Clinics of North America, 23*(2), 529–549.

Eisenberg, D. M., Kessler, R. C., Foster, C., Norlock, F. E., Calkins, D. R., & Delbanco, T. L. (1993). Unconventional medicine in the United States: Prevalence, costs, and patterns of use. New *England Journal of Medicine, 328,* 246-52.

French, S. D., Cameron, M., Walker, B. F., Reggars, J. W., & Esterman, A. J. (2006). Superficial heat or cold for low back pain. *Cochrane Database for Systemic Reviews, 2006* (2).

Furlan, A. D., Brosseau, L., Imamura, M., & Irvin, E. (2006). Massage for low back pain. *Cochrane Database for Systematic Reviews, 2006*(2).

Khatta, M. (2007). A complementary approach to pain management. *Topics in Advanced Practice Nursing eJournal, 7*(1). Retrieved 30 May 2007 from http://www.medscape.com/view-article/556408

National Center for Complementary and Alternative Medicine (NCCAM). (2004). *Expanding horizons of health care strategic plan 2005–2009.* Bethesda, MD: U.S. Department of Health and Human Services, National Institutes of Health.

O'Hara, D. A. (2003). Pain management. In P. Iyer (Ed.), *Medical legal aspects of suffering.* Tucson, AZ: Lawyers and Judges Publishing.

Pierce, B. (2009). A nonpharmacologic adjunct for pain management. *The Nurse Practitioner, 34*(2), 10-13.

CHAPTER 5

American Pain Society (APS). (2009). *Principles of analgesic use in the treatment of acute pain and cancer pain.* Glenview, IL: The Society.

American Society for Pain Management Nursing (ASPMN). (2006). Position statement: Authorized and unauthorized ("PCA by proxy") dosing of analgesic infusion pumps. Retrieved from http://www.aspmn.org/Organization/documents/PCAbyProxy-final-EW_004.pdf

American Society of Perianesthesia Nurses (ASPAN). (2003). Pain and comfort clinical guidelines. *Journal of Perianesthesia Nursing, 18*(4), 232–236.

Ashburn, M., Caplan, R., Carr, D., Connis, R., Ginsberg, B., Green, C., et al. (2004). Practice guidelines for acute pain management in the perioperative setting. *Anesthesiology, 100*(6), 1–15.

Clayton, J. (2008). Special needs of older adults undergoing surgery. *AORN, 87*(3), 557-574.

Cohen, M. (2006). *Patient controlled analgesia: Making it safer for patients.* Retrieved 22 November 2005 from http://www.ismp.org/profdevelopment/PCAMonograph.pdf

Cohen, M., & Smetzer, J. (2005). Patient-controlled analgesia safety issues. *Journal of Pain and Palliative Care Pharmcotherapy,19*(1), 45-50.

Cordell, W.H., Keene, K.K., Giles, B.K., Jones, J.B., Jones, J.H., & Brizendine, E.J. (2002). The high prevalence of pain in emergency care. *American Journal of Emergency Medicine*, *20*(3), 165-169.

D'Arcy, Y. (2007). *Pain management: Evidence-based tools and techniques for nursing professionals*. Marblehead, MS: HcPro.

Gray-Vickrey, P. (2005). What's behind acute delirium? *Nursing made incredibly easy*, *3*(1), 20-28.

Horgas, A., McLennon, S., & Floetke, A. (2003). Pain management in persons with dementia. *Alzheimer's Care*, *4*(4), 297-311.

Huffman, J., & Kunik, M. (2000). Assessment and understanding of pain in patients with dementia. *The Gerontologist*, *40*(5), 574-581.

Idelli, P. F, Grant, S., Neilsen, K., & Parker, T. (2005). Regional anesthesia in hip surgery. *Clinical Orthopedics and Related Research*, *441*, 250-255.

Inouye, S., Van Dyk, C. H., Alessi, C. A., Balkin, S., Siegal, A. P., & Horwitz, R. (1990). *Annals of Internal Medicine*, *113*, 941-948.

Joint Commission on Accreditation of Healthcare Organizations. (2000). *Pain assessment and management: An organizational approach*. Oakbrook Terrace, IL: JCAHO.

Karani, R., & Meier, D. (2004). Systematic pharmacologic postoperative pain management in the geriatric orthopedic patient. *Clinical Orthopedics and Related Research*, *425*, 26-34.

Liu, S., & Salinas, F. V. (2003). Continuous plexus and peripheral nerve blocks for postoperative analgesia. *Anesthesia and Analgesia*, *96*(1), 263-272.

Singer, A. J., Richman, P. B., Kowalska, A., & Thode, H. C. (1999.) Comparison of patient and practitioner assessments of pain from commonly performed emergency department procedures. *Annals of Emergency Medicine*, *33*(6), 652-658.

Vaurio, L., Sands, L., Wang, Y., Mullen, E. A., & Leung, J. (2006). Postoperative delirium: The importance of pain and pain management. *Anesthesia & Analgesia*, *102*(4), 1267-1273.

CHAPTER 6

Abrams, D., Jay, C., Shade, S., Vizoso, H., Reda, H., Press, S., et al. (2007). Cannabis in painful HIV associated sensory neuropathy: A randomized placebo controlled trial. *Neurology*, *68*(7), 515-521.

American Geriatrics Society, Panel on Persistent Pain in Older Persons. (2002). The management of persistent pain in older persons. *Journal of the American Geriatrics Society*, *50*, S205-S224.

American Health Care Association. (n.d.). *Nursing home statistics (AHCA)*. Retrieved 4 April 2009 from http://www.efmoody.com/longterm/nursingstatistics.html

American Pain Society. (2002). *Pain in osteoarthritis, rheumatoid arthritis, and juvenile chronic arthritis*. Glenview, IL: Author.

American Pain Society. (2005). *Pain control in the primary care setting*. Glenview, IL: Author.

American Society for Pain Management Nursing. (2002). *Core curriculum for pain management nursing*. Philadelphia: W.B. Saunders.

Bruckenthal, P., & D'Arcy, Y. (2007). Assessment and management of pain in older adults: A review of the basics. *Topics in Advanced Practice Nursing eJournal*, *7*(1). Retrieved 4 April 2009 from http://www.medscape.com/viewarticle

Buffum, M., Miaskowski, C., & Sands, L. (2001). A pilot study of the relationship between discomfort and agitation in patients with dementia. *Geriatric Nursing*, *22*(2), 80-85.

Cayea, D. (2006). Chronic low back pain in older adults: What physicians should know, what they think they know, and what they should be taught. *Journal of the American Geriatrics Society*, *53*(11), 1772-1777.

Centers for Disease Control and Prevention. (2007). Diabetes Public Health Resource. Retrieved 22 November 2009 from http://cdc.gov/diabetes.

Chou, R., & Huffman, L. (2007). Medications for acute and low back pain: A review of the evidence for an American Pain Society/American College of Physicians Clinical Practice Guideline. *Annals of Internal Medicine*, *147*(7), 505-514.

Chou, R., Qaseem, A., Snow, V., Casey, D., Cross, J.T., Shekelle, P., et al. (2007). Diagnosis and treatment of low back pain: A joint clinical practice guideline from the American College of Physicians and American Pain Society. *Annals of Internal Medicine*, *147*(7), 478-491.

D'Arcy, Y. (2007). *Pain management: Evidence based tools and techniques for nursing professionals.* Marblehead, MA: HcPro.

D'Arcy, Y. (2008a). Pain in the older adult. *The Nurse Practitioner, 33*(3), 19-25.

D'Arcy, Y. (2008b). Difficult to treat chronic pain syndromes. *The Clinical Advisor*, 27-34.

D'Arcy, Y. (2009). Is low back pain getting on your nerves? *The Nurse Practitioner, 34*(5), 17-18.

Davies, P., & Galer, B.(2004). Review of lidocaine patch 5% studies in the treatment of postherpetic neuralgia. *Drugs, 64*(9), 937-947.

Eichenberger, U., Neff, F., Sveticic, G., Bjorgo, S., Petersen-Felix, S., Arendt-Nielsen, L., et al. (2008). Chronic phantom limb pain: The effects of calcitonin, ketamine, and their combination on pain and sensory thresholds. *Anesthesia & Analgesia, 106*(4), 1265-1273.

Dworkin, R. H., Corbin, A. E., Young, J. P., Sharma, U., LaMoreaux, M., Bockbrader, H., et al. (2003). Pregabalin for the treatment of postherpetic neuralgia: A randomized placebo controlled trial. *Neurology*, 60, 1274-1283.

Dworkin, R. H., O'Connor, A. B., Backonja, M., Farrar, J. T., Finnerup, N. P, Jensen T. S., et al. (2007). Pharmacological management of neuropathic pain: Evidence based recommendations. *Pain, 132*, 237-251.

Huffman, J., & Kunik, M. (2000). Assessment and understanding of pain in patients with dementia. *The Gerontologist, 40*(5), 574-581.

Hutt, E., Buffum, M., Fink, R., Jones, K., & Pepper, G. (2007). Optimizing pain management in long-term care residents. *Geriatrics Aging, 10*(8), 523-527.

Lin, E. H., Katon W., Von Korff, M., Tang, L., Williams, J. W. Jr., Kroenke, K., et al. (2003). IMPACT investigators. Effect of improving depression care on pain and functional outcomes among older adults with arthritis: A randomized controlled trial. *JAMA, 290*(18), 2428-2429.

Hampton, T. (2005). When shingles wanes but pain does not. *JAMA, 293*(20), 2459-2460.

Khaliq, W., Alam, S., & Puri, N. (2008). Topical lidocaine for the treatment of postherpetic neuralgia. *The Cochrane Database of Systematic Reviews, 1.*

LaGranga, M. L., & Monmanney, T. (2001, June 15). Doctor found liable in suit over pain. *The Los Angeles Times*, p. A1, A34.

Matthews, F., & Dening, T. (2002). Prevalence of dementia in institutional care. *The Lancet, 360*, 225-226.

Merskey, H., & Bogduk, N. (1994). Classification of chronic pain: Descriptions of chronic syndromes and definitions of pain terms. In H. Merskey & N. Bogduk N. (Eds.), *Task force on taxonomy of the International Association for the Study of Pain.* Seattle, WA: IASP Press.

Morantz, C., & Torrey, B. (2005). Practice guideline briefs. *American Family Physician*, *71*(4), 1-3.

National Institute for Health and Clinical Excellence. (2009). *Low Back Pain: Early Management of Persistent Non-Specific Low Back Pain*. London, England: The Institute.

Oxman, M. N., Levin, M. J, Johnson, G. R., Schamder, K. E., Straus, S. E., Gelb, L. D., et al. (2005). A vaccine to prevent herpes zoster and postherpetic neuralgia in older adults. *New England Journal of Medicine*, *352*(22), 2271-2284.

Pasero, C., & McCaffery, M. (2001). The undertreatment of pain. *American Journal of Nursing*, *101*(11), 62.

Polomano, R., & Farrar, J. (2006). Pain and neuropathy in cancer survivors. *Cancer Nursing*, *29*(2 Suppl), 39-47.

Reyes-Gibby, C. C., Aday, L. A., Todd, K. H., Cleeland, C. S., & Anderson, K. O. (2007). Pain in aging community dwelling adults in the United States: Non-hispanic whites, non-Hispanic blacks, and Hispanics. *Journal of Pain*, *8*, 75-84.

Sandy, M. (2005). Herpes zoster: Medical and nursing management. *Clinical Journal of Oncology Nursing*, *9*(4), 443-446.

Smeltzer, S., Bare, B., Hinkle, J., & Cheever, K. (2007). *Brunner and Suddarth's textbook of medical surgical nursing* (11th ed.). Philadelphia: Lippincott, Williams, and Wilkins.

Staats, P., Argoff, C., Brewer, R., D'Arcy, Y., Gallagher, R., McCarberg, W., et al. (2004). Neuropathic pain: Incorporating new consensus guidelines into the reality of clinical practice. *Advanced Studies in Medicine*, *4*(78). Retrieved 4 April 2009 from http://www.JHASIM.com

Valente, S. (2008). Suicide risk in elderly patients. *The Nurse Practitioner*, *33*(8), 34-40.

Varela-Burstein, E., & Miller, P. (2003). Is chronic pain a risk factor for falls among community dwelling elders? *Topics in Geriatric Rehabilitation*, *19*(2), 145-159.

Wallace, A., & Wallace, M. (1997). Pain: Nociceptive and neuropathic mechanisms. *Anesthesia Clinics of North America*, *15*(2), 1-17.

Wernicke, J. F., Pritchett, Y. L., D'Souza, D. N., Waninger, A., Tran, P., Iyengar, S., et al. (2006). A randomized controlled trial of duloxetine in diabetic peripheral neuropathic pain. *Neurology*, *67*, 1411-1420.

Yi, M. (2001, June 15). Doctor found reckless for not relieving pain. *San Francisco Chronicle*, p. A1, A18.

CHAPTER 7

American Pain Society. (2006). Managing pain in primary care. Glenview, IL: American Pain Society.

Armon, C., Argoff, C., Samuels, J., & Backonja, M. (2007). Assessment: Use of epidural steroid injections to treat radicular lumbosacral pain: Report of the Therapeutics and Technology Assessment Subcommittee of the American Academy of Neurology. *Neurology*, *68*(10), 723-729.

Barclay, L., & Lie, D. (2008). Calcium supplementation may reduce fracture risk. *Medscape*. Retrieved 1 June 2008 from http://www.medscape.com/viewarticle/576008

Chou, R., & Huffman, L. (2007). Medications for acute and chronic low back pain: A review of evidence for an American Pain Society/American College of Physicians Clinical Practice Guideline. *Annals of Internal Medicine*, *147*(7), 505-514.

Dagenais, S., Yelland, M., Del Ma, C., & Schoene, M. (2009). Prolotherapy injections for chronic low back pain, *Cochrane Database for Systematic Reviews, 3*.

Freeman, B., Fraser, R., Cain, C., Hall, D., & Chappie, D. (2005). A randomized, double blind, controlled trial: Intradiscal electrothermal therapy versus placebo for the treatment of chronic discogenic low back pain. *Spine, 30*(21), 2369-2377.

Hulme, P. A., Krebs, J., Ferguson, S., & Berlemann, U. (2006). Vertebroplasty and kyphoplasty: A systematic review of 69 clinical studies, *Spine, 31*(17), 1983-2001.

Kessenich, C. (2003). PTH revisited for osteoporosis treatment. *The Nurse Practitioner, 28*(6), 51-53.

Lynch, S. S., Cheng, C. M., & Yee, J. L. (2006). Intrathecal ziconotide for refractory chronic pain. *Annals of Pharmacotherapy, 40*(7-8), 1293-1200.

Mailis-Gagnon, A., Furlan, A., Sandoval, J. A., & Taylor, R. (2008). Spinal cord stimulation for chronic pain. *The Cochrane Database of Systemic Reviews, 3*.

Manheimer, E., White, A., Berman, B., Forys, K., & Ernst, E. (2005). Meta-analysis: Acupuncture for low back pain. *Annals of Internal Medicine, 142*(8), 651-663.

National Institutes of Health, Osteoporosis and Related Bone Diseases National Resources Center. (n.d.) *Medications to prevent and treat osteoporosis*. Retrieved 1 April 2008 from http://www.niams.nih.gov/bone

Nelemans, P. J., deBie, R. A., deVet, H. C., & Sturmans, F. (2000). Injection therapy for subacute and chronic benign low back pain. Cochrane Review. *ACP Journal, 133*(1), 27.

NTAC (Neuromodulation Therapy Access Coalition). (2008). *Position statement on spinal cord neuromodulation*. Retrieved 1 April 2008 from http://www.aapm.org

Phillips, F. (2003) Minimally invasive treatments of osteoporotic vertebral compression fractures. *Spine, 28*(15S), S45-S53.

Prince, R., Devine, A., Sarvinder, S., & Dick, I. (2006). Effects of calcium supplementation on clinical fracture and bone structure. *Archives of Internal Medicine, 166*(8), 869-875.

Schroeder, C. I., Doering, C. J., Zamponi, G. W., & Lewis, R. J. (2006). N-type calcium channel blockers: Novel therapeutics for the treatment of pain. *Medicinal Chemistry, 2*(5), 535-543.

Smeltzer, S., Bare, B., Hinkle, J., & Cheever, K. (2007). *Brunner & Suddarth's textbook of medical surgical nursing* (11th ed.). Philadelphia: Lippincott Williams & Wilkins.

Wallace, M., & Staats, P. (2005). *Pain medicine and management*. New York: McGraw-Hill.

CHAPTER 8

Aging with Dignity. (2009). *Five wishes*. Retrieved 10 November 2009 from http://www.agingwithdignity.org/5wishes.html

Beck, A., Steer, R., & Carbin, M. (1988). Psychometric properties of the Beck Depression Index: Twenty-five years of evaluation. *Clinical Psychology Review, 8*(1), 77-100.

Brown, P., Woods, C., & Storandt, M. (2007). Model stability of the 15 item Geriatric Depression Scale across cognitive impairment and severe depression. *Psychology and Aging, 22*(2), 372-379.

Buntin-Mushock, C., Phillip, L., Moriyama, K., & Palmer, P. P. (2005). Age dependent opioid escalations in chronic pain patients. *Anesthesia & Analgesia, 100*, 1740-1745.

D'Arcy, Y. (2007). One pain medication does not fit all: Using opioid rotation in your practice. *The Nurse Practitioner, 32*(11), 7-8.

Health Promotion Board. *Strong bones for life.* Retrieved 11 November 2009 from http://hpb.gov.sg/data/hpb.home/files/pro/strongbonesforlife_e_.pdf

Indelicato, R. A., Portnoy, R. (2002). Opioid rotation in the management of refractory cancer pain. *Journal of Clinical Oncology, 20*(1), 348-352.

Kuebler, K., Berry, P., & Heidrich, D. (2002). *End of life care: Clinical practice guidelines.* Philadelphia: W.B. Saunders Co.

Long, J. D., Harring, J. H., Brekke, J. S., Test, M. A., & Greenberg, J. (2007). Longitudinal construct validity of the Brief Symptom Inventory subscales in schizophrenia. *Psychological Assessment, 19*(3), 298-308.

McLennon, S. M. (2005). *Persistent pain management.* University of Iowa Gerontological Nursing Interventions Research Center. Retrieved 9 November 2009 from http://www.guideline.gov/summary/summary.aspx?doc_id=8627&nbr=004807&string=persistent+AND+pain+AND+management

Mercandante, S., & Bruera, E. (2006). Opioid switching: A systematic and critical review. *Cancer Treatment Reviews, 32*, 302-315.

Oncology Watch. (2002, 2003). The Advisory Board. Retrieved 1 April 2008 from http://www.Advisoryboard.com

Qaseem, A., Snow, V., Shekeele, P., Casey, D. E., Cross, J. T., & Owens, D. K. (2008). *Evidence-based interventions to improve the palliative care of pain, dyspnea, and depression at the end of life: A clinical practice guideline from the American College of Physicians.* National Guideline Clearing House. Retrieved 1 April 2009 from http://www.guideline.gov

Quigley, C. (2006). Opioid switching to improve pain relief and drug tolerability. *The Cochrane Database of Systemic Reviews, 4.*

Smeltzer, S., Bare, B., Hinkle, J., & Cheever, K. (2008). *Brunner & Suddarth's textbook of medical surgical nursing* (11th ed.). Philadelphia: Lippincott Williams & Wilkins.

Whitecar, P. S., Maxwell, T. L., & Douglass, A.B. (2004). Principles of palliative care medicine: Part 2: Pain and symptom management. *Advanced Studies in Medicine, 4*(2), 88-100.

World Health Organization. (1990). In S. Smeltzer, B. Bare, J. Hinkle, & K. Cheever, 2008, *Brunner & Suddarth's textbook of medical surgical nursing* (11th ed.). Philadelphia: Lippincott Williams & Wilkins.

INDEX

A

absorption of medications, physiology and, 6
acetaminophen, 43, 106
active listening (nurse's role), 160
acupuncture, 66–67, 123
acute low back pain, 105
acute pain
  assessment, 15–18
  management
    case study, 92–93
    delirium/dementia, 89–92
    emergency department, 80–82
    older patients, 78–79
    postoperative pain, 84–89
    surgical area, 82–84
addiction, opioids and, 48–49
advance directives, 148–149
aggravating factors (pain assessment), 14
aging of America, 1–9
Aging With Dignity, 148
AGS (American Geriatrics Society) paper (2002), 2–4, 26, 33, 62, 67–69, 115
alleviating factors (pain assessment), 14
American Geriatrics Society (AGS) paper (2002), 2
American Pain Society (APS), 105
American Society of Anesthesiologists, 87

American Society of PeriAnesthesia Nurses (ASPAN), 84–85
amitriptyline, 52
anesthesia, 88-89
anticonvulsants, 53
antidepressants, 53, 110, 158
anxiolytics (respiratory distress management), 151
anxiety, 158–159
APS (American Pain Society), 105, 125
Arthritis Self-Management Program (ASMP), 69, 103
ASMP (Arthritis Self-Management Program), 69, 103
ASPAN (American Society of PeriAnesthesia Nurses), 84–85
assessment of pain, 11
  acute pain, 15–18, 78-79
  basic elements, 12–15
  case study, 31–32
  chronic pain, 18–24
  nonverbal patients, 25–30
Avinza, 50
axial pain, 104

B

basic elements, pain assessment, 12–15
BDI (Beck Depression Inventory), 157

Beck Depression Inventory (BDI), 157
behavioral indicators, 25–26
binding ability, opioids, 47
biofeedback, 70
body-based CAM therapies, 64–68
bone
    normal versus osteoporotic, 134
    pain, 153
BPI (Brief Pain Inventory), 19, 22–23
BPIQ (Brief Pain Impact Questionnaire), 19, 24
breakthrough pain, 55
Brief Pain Impact Questionnaire (BPIQ), 19, 24
Brief Pain Inventory (BPI), 19, 22–23
Brief Symptom Inventory (BSI), 158
bronchodilators (respiratory distress management), 151
BSI (Brief Symptom Inventory), 158

C

CAM (complementary and alternative medicine)
    body-based therapies, 64–68
    case study, 74–75
    cognitive behavioral therapy, 68–70
    energy therapies, 70–72
    nutritional approaches, 72–73
    types of, 63–64
Capsaicin cream, 54
Capsicum (herbal remedy), 72–73
cardiovascular risks, NSAIDs, 45–46
care team (palliative care), 145–147
case studies
    acute pain management, 92–93
    chronic pain management, 119–120
    complementary and alternative medicine, 74–75
    interventional pain management, 141–142
    medication management, 58–60
    pain assessment, 31–32
    palliative care, 161–163
    problem-solving pain management issues, 8–9

categories
    low back pain, 105
    older patients, 2–3
cayenne (herbal remedy), 72–73
characteristics of chronic pain, 99–101
Checklist of Nonverbal Pain Indicators (CNPI), 25
chemotherapy-related neuropathies, 113–114
chiropractic therapy, 67
chondroitin, 73
chronic pain
    assessment, 18–24
    common conditions, 96
    low back pain (LBP), 104–107
    management, 95
        case study, 119–120
        characteristics of pain, 99–101
        long-term care, 114–118
        low back pain, 104–107
        neuropathic pain syndromes, 107–114
        osteoarthritis, 101–104
        undertreatment, 97–99
    presentations, 100
CNPI (Checklist of Nonverbal Pain Indicators), 25
coanalgesics, 53–54
The Cochrane Collaboration, 65
Cochrane Database of Systematic Reviews, 65
codeine, 49
cognitive behavioral therapy, 68–70
cognitively impaired patients
    myths about pain, 5
    pain assessment, 14
cold and heat (body-based CAM therapy), 64–66
comfort care physician orders, 155–156
complex regional pain syndrome (CRPS), 15, 107
compression fractures, osteoporosis, 133–140
    comparison of bone, 134
    kyphosis, 133, 135
    patient education, 137
    risks, 136–137
    treatment options, 137–138
constipation, 56

contraindications, SCS (spinal cord stimulation), 132
Corydalis (herbal remedy), 73
COX-2 selective NSAIDs, 44
CRPS (complex regional pain syndrome), 15, 107
curative care versus palliative care, 144
CYP450 (cytochrome P450) system, opioid metabolism, 47

D

Darvocet, 52
Darvon, 52
DDD (degenerative disc disease), 104, 123
definitions
    acute pain, 15
    aging, 1
    CAM (complementary and alternative medicine), 62
    delirium, 89
    dementia, 90
    kyphoplasty, 139
    opioid naive, 47
    opioid tolerance, 47
    polypharmacy, 38
    vertebroplasty, 139
degenerative disc disease (DDD), 104, 123
delirium, acute pain management, 89–92
dementia
    acute pain management, 89–92
    pain and, 115–117
Demerol, 52
depression management, 102-105, 157–158
description (pain assessment), 13–14
Devil's claw (herbal remedy), 73
diabetic neuropathy, 108–111
Dietary Supplement Health and Education Act (DSHEA), 72
Dilaudid, 50–51
distribution of medications, physiology and, 6–7
Dolophine, 51

dose escalation, opioids, 152
DSHEA (Dietary Supplement Health and Education Act), 72
Duragesic patches, 51
duration (pain assessment), 13

E

education, osteoporosis, 137
Elavil, 52
elements of pain assessment, 12–15
elimination of medications, physiology and, 7
elite old category, 2
emergency department, acute pain management, 80–82
emesis, 56
energy CAM therapies, 70–72
enteral feeding devices, 154
epidural analgesia, 88
epiduroscopy, 126
ethnicity, opioid metabolism and, 47
excretion of medications, physiology and, 7
extended-release Vicodin, 49

F

Faces, Legs, Activity, Cry, Consolability (FLACC) scale, 27–28
failed back syndrome, 124
fall risks, 81–82
FDA (Food and Drug Administration), NSAIDs research, 44
Fentanyl, 51
Fentanyl Oralets, 51
Fentora, 51
Five Wishes advanced directive, 148
FLACC (Faces, Legs, Activity, Cry, Consolability) scale, 27–28
Food and Drug Administration (FDA), NSAIDs research, 44
Forteo (Teriperatide), 137–138
functional impairment, 14

G

gastrointestinal risks, NSAIDs, 44–45
gastrostomy tubes, 154
GDS (Geriatric Depression Scale), 157
Geriatric Depression Scale (GDS), 157
glucosamine, 73
goals of pain assessment, 14
good death, palliative care, 159–160

H

Harpagophytum procumbens (herbal remedy), 73
heat and cold (body-based CAM therapy), 64–66
herbal remedies, 72–73
hydrocodone/APAP, 49
hydromorphone, 50–51
hypnosis, 70

I

IASP (International Society for the Study of Pain), 107
IDET (intradiscal electrothermal therapy), 126
imagery (cognitive behavioral therapy), 69–70
implanted interventional modalities, 127–130
indicators of pain, nonverbal patients, 25–26
Indocin, 52
indomethacin, 52
injection techniques, interventional pain management, 125–126
Institute for Safe Medication Practices (ISMP), 86–87
integrative medicine, 64
intensity (pain assessment), 13
International Society for the Study of Pain (IASP), 107
interventional pain management, 121–142
    acupuncture, 123

case study, 141–142
implanted modalities, 126–130
modalities, 123–126
osteoporotic compression fractures, 133–140
spinal cord stimulation, 130–132
intradiscal electrothermal therapy (IDET), 126
intraoperative blocks, 88
intrathecal pumps, 127–130
ISMP (Institute for Safe Medication Practices), 86–87

J

JCAHO (Joint Commission on Accreditation of Healthcare Organizations), pain management standards, 79
joints, osteoarthritis pain, 102

K

Kadian, 50
Krieger, Dolores, 71
Kunz, Dora, 71
kyphoplasty, 138–140
kyphosis, 135

L

LBP (low back pain), 104–107
LFTs (liver function tests), 43
lidocaine patches, 54
Lidoderm Patch 5%, 54
liver function tests (LFTs), 43
local anesthesia pumps, 89
location (pain assessment), 13
long-term care, 114–118
Lortab, 49
low back pain (LBP), 104–107

M

management
    acute pain
        case study, 92–93
        delirium/dementia, 89–92

emergency department, 80–82
  older patients, 78–79
  postoperative pain, 84–89
  surgical area, 82–84
chronic pain, 95–120
  case study, 119–120
  characteristics of pain, 99–101
  long-term care, 114–118
  low back pain, 104–107
  neuropathic pain syndromes, 107–114
  osteoarthritis, 101–104
  undertreatment, 97–99
palliative care, 149–159
  physical symptoms, 149–156
  psychosocial symptoms, 157–159
massage, 67
McGill Pain Questionnaire (MPQ), 19–21
medication management
  anxiety treatment, 159
  appetite stimulation, 154
  breakthrough pain, 55
  case study, 58–60
  coanalgesics, 53–54
  influence of physiology, 6–7
  intrathecal pumps, 127–130
  mild pain, 42
    acetaminophen, 43
    NSAIDs, 43–46
  neuropathic pain, 110–111
  nonverbal patients, 39–40
  nursing considerations, 57–58
  opioids
    mild pain, 46–52
    moderate pain, 49–50
    myths about pain, 4–5
    severe pain, 50–51
  selecting the right medication, 41–57
  side effects, 55–57
  special considerations, 37–40
  topical analgesics, 54–55
  use of medications in older patients, 36–37
meditation, 70
meperidine, 52
metabolism (medications), 6–7, 47
Methadone, 51

mild pain
  medication management, 42–46
    acetaminophen, 43
    NSAIDs, 43–46
    opioids, 46–52
  WHO (World Health Organization) ladder, 41–42
mind-body work, 68–70
modalities, interventional pain management, 123–126
moderate pain
  medication management, 49–50
  WHO (World Health Organization) ladder, 41–42
modified FLACC scale, 27–28
morphine, 50, 150
Morphine IR, 50
MPQ (McGill Pain Questionnaire), 19–21
MS Contin, 50
multilevel plans of care, low back pain, 106–107
myths about pain, 3–6

N

naive (opioid use) persons, 47
National Center for Complementary and Alternative Medicine (NCCAM), 61
nausea, 56
NCCAM (National Center for Complementary and Alternative Medicine), 61
NDRI (norepinephrine-dopamine reuptake inhibitor), 158
neuronal-type (N-type) calcium channel blockers, Ziconotide, 128–129
neuropathic pain syndromes, 107–114, 153
nociceptive pain, 108
nonselective NSAIDs, 44
nonspecific low back pain, 105
nonsteroidal anti-inflammatory drugs. See NSAIDs
nonverbal patients
  medication management, 39–40
  myths about pain, 5
  pain assessment, 25–30

norepinephrine-dopamine reuptake
  inhibitor (NDRI), 158
NRS (Numeric Pain Rating Scale),
  16
NSAIDs (nonsteroidal anti-
  inflammatory drugs), 33, 43–46
  cardiovascular risks, 45–46
  gastrointestinal risks, 44–45
  low back pain treatment, 106
  patches, 55
Numeric Pain Rating Scale (NRS),
  16
nurse's role, palliative care, 160–161
nutrition
  CAM approaches, 72–73
  management of physical
    symptoms, 153–156
  supplements, 73

O

OA (osteoarthritis), 101–104
older old category, 2
older patients, acute pain, 78–79
omega-3 fatty acids, 73
Opana, 50
Opana ER, 50
opioids
  addiction and, 48–49
  dose escalation, 152
  influence of physiology, 36
  low back pain treatment, 106
  medications to avoid, 51–52
  metabolism, 47
  moderate pain management,
    49–50
  myths about pain, 4–5
  neuropathic pain treatment, 110
  physical dependence, 49
  polymorphism, 46
  postoperative period, 85
  pseudo-addiction, 49
  rotation, 152
  severe pain management, 50–51
  tolerance, 49
  toxicity, 4
osteoarthritis (OA), 101–104
osteoporosis, 133–140
  comparison of bone, 134
  kyphosis, 135

patient education, 137
  risks, 136–137
  treatment options, 137–138
osteoporotic compression fractures.
  See osteoporosis
oxycodone/APAP, 49–50
Oxycontin, 49–50
Oxyfast, 49–50
oxymorphone, 50

P

Pain Assessment in Advanced
  Dementia (PAINAD) scale, 29–30
Pain/Distress Intensity Scale, 18
PAINAD (Pain Assessment in
  Advanced Dementia) scale, 29–30
painful diabetic neuropathy (PDN),
  108–111
palliative care, 143–163
  advance directives, 148–149
  care team, 145–147
  case study, 161–163
  good death, 159–160
  nurse's role, 160–161
  symptom management, 149–159
patient education, osteoporosis, 137
patient-controlled analgesia (PCA),
  86–87
PCA (patient-controlled analgesia),
  86–87
PDN (painful diabetic neuropathy),
  108–111
pentazocine, 52
Percocet, 49–50
Percodan, 49–50
pethidine, 52
PHN (postherpetic neuralgia),
  111–114
physical dependence, opioids, 49
Physical Performance Test (PPT), 19
physical symptom management,
  149–156
physical therapy, 67–68
physiology, medication use and, 6–7,
  36
placebos, 4
polypharmacy, 38–39
post-mastectomy pain syndrome,
  113–114

post-thoracotomy pain syndrome (PTPS), 113–114
post-treatment neuropathies, 113–114
postherpetic neuralgia (PHN), 111–113
postoperative pain, 84–89
PPI (present pain intensity) rating, 20
PPT (Physical Performance Test), 19
predictors, severe pain, 98
present pain intensity (PPI) rating, 20
problem-solving, 8–9
prolotherapy, 124, 126
propxyphene, 52
pruritis, 56
pseudo-addiction, opioids, 49
psychosocial symptom management, 157–159
PTPS (post-thoracotomy pain syndrome), 113

Q-R

radicular pain, 104-105, 124
radiculopathy, 105, 124
radiofrequency lesioning, 124, 126
referred pain, 104
relaxation (cognitive behavioral therapy), 68
reports of pain, 5–6
respiratory depression (side effect), 56
respiratory distress, 150–151
rest, ice, compression, and elevation (RICE) therapy, 66
RICE (rest, ice, compression, and elevation) therapy, 66
risks
    delirium, 90
    falls, 81–82
    implanted intrathecal pumps, 130
    mortality, 83–84
    osteoporosis, 136–137
    PHN (postherpetic neuralgia), 111–112
    surgical tolerance, 83
rotation, opioids, 152
Roxanol, 50

S

Salix alba (herbal remedy), 73
scales, pain evaluation/assessment
    BPI (Brief Pain Inventory), 19, 22–23
    BPIQ (Brief Pain Impact Questionnaire), 19, 24
    FLACC (Faces, Legs, Activity, Cry, Consolability), 27–28
    MPQ (McGill Pain Questionnaire), 19–21
    NRS (Numeric Pain Rating Scale), 16
    PAINAD (Pain Assessment in Advanced Dementia), 29–30
    Thermometer Pain Scale, 18
    VDS (Verbal Descriptor Scale), 17
    Visual Analog Scale, 16–17
SCS (spinal cord stimulation), 130–132
sedation, 56
selective serotonin reuptake inhibitors (SSRIs), 53, 158
sensation of pain, 5
serotonin-norepinephrine reuptake inhibitors (SNRIs), 53-54, 158
severe pain
    medication management, 50–51
    predictors, 98
    WHO (World Health Organization) ladder, 41–42
short-acting pain medications, 85
side effects
    influence of physiology, 37
    medication management, 55–57
    Ziconotide, 127–129
SNRIs (serotonin-norepinephrine reuptake inhibitors), 53-54, 158
sources of pain, LBP (low back pain), 104
spinal cord stimulation (SCS), 130–132
spinal processes, 124
spinal stenosis, 124
SSRIs (selective serotonin reuptake inhibitors), 53, 158
Stepwise Pharmacological Management Plan, 109–110

steroids
  interventional pain management,
    125
  management of respiratory
    distress, 151
Study to Understand Prognoses and
  Preferences for Outcomes and
  Risks of Treatments (SUPPORT),
  143
supplemental oxygen, 150
supplements, 73
SUPPORT (Study to Understand
  Prognoses and Preferences
  for Outcomes and Risks of
  Treatments), 143
surgical area, acute pain
  management, 82–84
symptom management (palliative
  care), 149–159

T

Talwin, 52
targeted topical analgesics, 54–55
TCAs (tricyclic antidepressants), 53
techniques, interventional pain
  management, 121
Teriperatide (Forteo), osteoporosis
  treatment, 137–138
Therapeutic Touch (TT), 71–72
Thermometer Pain Scale, 18
thoughtful communication (nurse's
  role), 160
tolerance, opioids, 47, 49
topical analgesics, 54–55
toxicity, opioids, 4
tramadol, 50
  low back pain treatment, 106
  neuropathic pain treatment, 111
treatments
  anxiety, 159
  depression, 158
  long-term care, 117–118
  low back pain, 105–107
  osteoarthritis pain, 103
  osteoporosis, 137–138
  painful diabetic neuropathy
    (PDN), 109–111
  PHN (postherpetic neuralgia),
    112–113

tricyclic antidepressants (TCAs), 53
trigger point injections, 125–126
TT (Therapeutic Touch), 71–72
Tylenol #3, 49

U

Ultracet, 50
Ultram, 50
Ultram ER, 50
undertreated pain, 2–3, 35
  chronic pain, 97–99
  consequences, 97
untreated pain, 2–3, 35
Usui, Mikao, 70

V

VDS (Verbal Descriptor Scale), 17
Verbal Descriptor Scale (VDS), 17
vertebroplasty, 138–140
Vicodin, 49
Visual Analog Scale, 16–17
vomiting, 56

W

WHO (World Health Organization)
  ladder, 41–42
willow bark (herbal remedy), 73
World Health Organization (WHO)
  ladder, 41–42

X-Y-Z

younger old category, 2

Ziconotide, 128–129
Zostrix, 54